Genetics and Precision Medicine

Editor

HOWARD P. LEVY

MEDICAL CLINICS
OF NORTH AMERICA

www.medical.theclinics.com

Consulting Editor
BIMAL H. ASHAR

November 2019 • Volume 103 • Number 6

ELSEVIER

1600 John F. Kennedy Boulevard • Suite 1800 • Philadelphia, Pennsylvania, 19103-2899

http://www.theclinics.com

MEDICAL CLINICS OF NORTH AMERICA Volume 103, Number 6
November 2019 ISSN 0025-7125, ISBN-13: 978-0-323-69625-8

Editor: Katerina Heidhausen
Developmental Editor: Kristen Helm

Medical Clinics of North America (ISSN 0025-7125) is published bimonthly by Elsevier Inc., 360 Park Avenue South, New York, NY 10010-1710. Months of publication are January, March, May, July, September, and November. Business and editorial offices: 1600 John F. Kennedy Boulevard, Suite 1800, Philadelphia, PA 19103-2899. Periodicals postage paid at New York, NY, and additional mailing offices. Subscription prices are USD $284.00 per year (US individuals), $611.00 per year (US institutions), $100.00 per year (US Students), $353.00 per year (Canadian individuals), $794.00 per year (Canadian institutions), $200.00 per year (Canadian and foreign students), $406.00 per year (foreign individuals), and $794.00 per year (foreign institutions). To receive student/resident rate, orders must be accompanied by name of affiliated institution, date of term, and the signature of program/residency coordinator on institution letterhead. Orders will be billed at individual rate until proof of status is received. Foreign air speed delivery is included in all Clinics' subscription prices. All prices are subject to change without notice. **POSTMASTER:** Send address changes to *Medical Clinics of North America*, Elsevier Health Sciences Division, Subscription Customer Service, 3251 Riverport Lane, Maryland Heights, MO 63043. **Customer Service: Telephone: 1-800-654-2452** (U.S. and Canada); **1-314-447-8871** (outside U.S. and Canada). **Fax: 314-447-8029. E-mail: journalscustomerserviceusa@elsevier.com** (for print support); **journalsonlinesupport-usa@elsevier.com** (for online support).

Reprints. For copies of 100 or more of articles in this publication, please contact the Commercial Reprints Department, Elsevier Inc., 360 Park Avenue South, New York, NY 10010-1710. Tel.: 212-633-3874; Fax: 212-633-3820; E-mail: reprints@elsevier.com.

Medical Clinics of North America is also published in Spanish by McGraw-Hill Interamericana Editores S. A., P.O. Box 5-237, 06500 Mexico, D.F., Mexico.

Medical Clinics of North America is covered in *MEDLINE/PubMed (Index Medicus), Current Contents, ASCA, Excerpta Medica, Science Citation Index, and ISI/BIOMED.*

PROGRAM OBJECTIVE
The goal of the *Medical Clinics of North America* is to keep practicing physicians up to date with current clinical practice by providing timely articles reviewing the state of the art in patient care.

TARGET AUDIENCE
All practicing physicians and other healthcare professionals.

LEARNING OBJECTIVES
Upon completion of this activity, participants will be able to:
1. Review how patient family medical history can inform differential diagnosis, risk assessment, and preventive counselling.
2. Discuss genetic testing in the assessment of Parkinson Disease.
3. Recognize clinical features, diagnostic work-up, and management of Neurofibromatosis Type1.

ACCREDITATION
The Elsevier Office of Continuing Medical Education (EOCME) is accredited by the Accreditation Council for Continuing Medical Education (ACCME) to provide continuing medical education for physicians.

The EOCME designates this journal-based CME activity for a maximum of 9 *AMA PRA Category 1 Credit*(s)™. Physicians should claim only the credit commensurate with the extent of their participation in the activity.

All other healthcare professionals requesting continuing education credit for this enduring material will be issued a certificate of participation.

DISCLOSURE OF CONFLICTS OF INTEREST
The EOCME assesses conflict of interest with its instructors, faculty, planners, and other individuals who are in a position to control the content of CME activities. All relevant conflicts of interest that are identified are thoroughly vetted by EOCME for fair balance, scientific objectivity, and patient care recommendations. EOCME is committed to providing its learners with CME activities that promote improvements or quality in healthcare and not a specific proprietary business or a commercial interest.

The planning committee, staff, authors and editors listed below have identified no financial relationships or relationships to products or devices they or their spouse/life partner have with commercial interest related to the content of this CME activity:
Bimal H. Ashar, MD, MBA, FACP; Robin L. Bennett, MS, CGC; Robert S. Brown Jr, MD, MPH; Curtis R. Coghlin II, MS, MBe, CGC; Erin Demo, MS, CGC; W. Andrew Faucett, MS, LGC; Madeline Graf, MS, LCGC; Patrick R. Heck, PhD; Katerina Heidhausen; Peter J. Hulick, MD, MMSc, FACMG; Nadim Ilbawi, MD; Alison Kemp; K. Ina Ly, MD; Gretchen MacCarrick, MS, CGC; Michelle N. Meyer, PhD, JD; Mitchel Pariani, MS, LCGC; Katelyn Payne, RN, CGC; Holly Peay, MS, PhD, CGC; Andrea L. Rideout, MS, CCGC, CGC; Emily A. Schonfeld, MD; Jeyanthi Surendrakumar; Dyson T. Wake, PharmD; Brooke Walls, MD

The planning committee, staff, authors and editors listed below have identified financial relationships or relationships to products or devices they or their spouse/life partner have with commercial interest related to the content of this CME activity:
Jaishri O. Blakeley, MD is a consultant/advisor for AbbVie Inc., AstraZeneca, Exelixis, Inc., and SpringWorks Therapeutics; receives research support from GlaxoSmithKline plc, ImClone Systems Incorporated, and Sanofi-Aventis U.S. LLC.
Henry M. Dunnenberger, PharmD is a consultant/advisor for Admera Health and Veritas

Howard P. Levy, MD, PhD is a consultant/advisor for eviCore Healthcare

Ellen Regalado, MS, CGC holds stock in Invitae Corporation

Christina Rigelsky, MS, CGC is a consultant/advisor for My Gene Counsel

Brad T. Tinkle, MD, PhD is a consultant/advisor for Resolys Bio, Inc. and serves on speakers bureau for Alexion Pharmaceuticals, Inc.

Joanne Wojcieszek, MD receives research support from Vaccinex Inc.

UNAPPROVED/OFF-LABEL USE DISCLOSURE
The EOCME requires CME faculty to disclose to the participants;
1. When products or procedures being discussed are off-label, unlabelled, experimental, and/or investigational (not US Food and Drug Administration [FDA] approved); and

2. Any limitations on the information presented, such as data that are preliminary or that represent ongoing research, interim analyses, and/or unsupported opinions. Faculty may discuss information about pharmaceutical agents that is outside of FDA-approved labelling. This information is intended solely for CME and is not intended to promote off-label use of these medications. If you have any questions, contact the medical affairs department of the manufacturer for the most recent prescribing information.

TO ENROLL
To enroll in the *Medical Clinics of North America* Continuing Medical Education program, call customer service at 1-800-654-2452 or sign up online at http://www.theclinics.com/home/cme. The CME program is available to subscribers for an additional annual fee of USD $300.90.

METHOD OF PARTICIPATION
In order to claim credit, participants must complete the following;
1. Complete enrolment as indicated above.
2. Read the activity.
3. Complete the CME Test and Evaluation. Participants must achieve a score of 70% on the test. All CME Tests and Evaluations must be completed online.

CME INQUIRIES/SPECIAL NEEDS
For all CME inquiries or special needs, please contact elsevierCME@elsevier.com.

MEDICAL CLINICS OF NORTH AMERICA

SERIES OF RELATED INTEREST

Primary Care: Clinics in Office Practice
Available at: http://www.primarycare.theclinics.com
Physician Assistant Clinics
Available at: http://www.physicianassistant.theclinics.com

Geriatric and Palliative Medicine

MEDICAL CLINICS OF NORTH AMERICA

FORTHCOMING ISSUES

January 2020
Allergy and Immunology for the Internist
Anne M. Ditto, Editor

March 2020
Physical Medicine and Rehabilitation for the
Primary Care Internists
David A. Lenrow, Editor

May 2020
Palliative Care
Eric Widera, Editor

RECENT ISSUES

September 2019
Cardiac Arrhythmias & Resynchronization
Otto Costantini, Editor

July 2019
Women's Mental Health
Susan G. Kornstein and Anita H. Clayton, Editors

May 2019
Pulmonary Disease
Ali I. Musani, Editor

SERIES OF RELATED INTEREST

Primary Care: Clinics in Office Practice
Available at: http://www.primarycare.theclinics.com
Physician Assistant Clinics
Available at: https://www.physicianassistant.theclinics.com

Contributors

CONSULTING EDITOR

BIMAL H. ASHAR, MD, MBA, FACP
Associate Professor of Medicine, Division of General Internal Medicine, Johns Hopkins University School of Medicine, Baltimore, Maryland, USA

EDITOR

HOWARD P. LEVY, MD, PhD
Associate Professor, Division of General Internal Medicine, Department of Medicine, McKusick-Nathans Institute of Genetic Medicine, Johns Hopkins University, Baltimore, Maryland, USA

AUTHORS

ROBIN L. BENNETT, MS, CGC
Clinical Professor, Division of Medical Genetics, Department of Medicine, University of Washington, University of Washington Medical Center, Seattle, Washington, USA

JAISHRI O. BLAKELEY, MD
Departments of Neurology and Neurosurgery, and Oncology, Johns Hopkins University, Baltimore, Maryland, USA

ROBERT S. BROWN Jr, MD, MPH
Division of Gastroenterology and Hepatology, Weill Cornell Medical College, New York, New York, USA

CURTIS R. COUGHLIN II, MS, MBe, CGC
Associate Professor, Department of Pediatrics, Section of Genetics, University of Colorado Anschutz Medical Campus, Aurora, Colorado, USA

ERIN DEMO, MS, CGC
Sibley Heart Center Cardiology, Atlanta, Georgia, USA

HENRY MARK DUNNENBERGER, PharmD
Director, Pharmacogenomics, Mark R. Neaman Center for Personalized Medicine, NorthShore University HealthSystem, Evanston, Illinois, USA

W. ANDREW FAUCETT, MS, LGC
Professor, Office of the Chief Scientific Officer, Geisinger, Danville, Pennsylvania, USA

MADELINE GRAF, MS, LCGC
Stanford Health Care, Stanford, California, USA

PATRICK R. HECK, PhD
Postdoctoral Fellow, Autism & Developmental Medicine Institute, Geisinger, Lewisburg, Pennsylvania, USA; Center for Translational Bioethics and Health Care Policy, Geisinger, Danville, Pennsylvania, USA

PETER J. HULICK, MD, MMSc, FACMG
Division Head, Center for Medical Genetics, Medical Director, Mark R. Neaman Center for Personalized Medicine, NorthShore University HealthSystem, Clinical Assistant Professor, University of Chicago, Pritzker School of Medicine, Evanston, Illinois, USA

NADIM ILBAWI, MD
Department of Family Medicine, NorthShore University HealthSystem, Lincolnwood, Illinois; Clinician Educator, University of Chicago, Pritzker School of Medicine, Chicago, Illinois, USA

HOWARD P. LEVY, MD, PhD
Associate Professor, Division of General Internal Medicine, Department of Medicine, McKusick-Nathans Institute of Genetic Medicine, Johns Hopkins University, Baltimore, Maryland, USA

K. INA LY, MD
Stephen E. and Catherine Pappas Center for Neuro-Oncology, Massachusetts General Hospital, Boston, Massachusetts, USA

GRETCHEN MacCARRICK, MS, CGC
Johns Hopkins School of Medicine, Baltimore, Maryland, USA

MICHELLE N. MEYER, PhD, JD
Assistant Professor and Associate Director, Research Ethics, Center for Translational Bioethics and Health Policy, Faculty-Co-Director, Behavioral Insights Team, Steele Institute for Innovation, Geisinger, Danville, Pennsylvania, USA

MITCHEL PARIANI, MS, LCGC
Stanford School of Medicine, Stanford, California, USA

KATELYN PAYNE, RN, CGC
Genetic Counselor, Department of Neurology, Indiana University School of Medicine, Indianapolis, Indiana, USA

HOLLY PEAY, MS, PhD, CGC
Senior Researcher, Center for Newborn Screening, Ethics, and Disability Studies, RTI International, Research Triangle Park, North Carolina, USA

ELLEN REGALADO, MS, CGC
Invitae, San Francisco, California, USA

ANDREA L. RIDEOUT, MS, CCGC, CGC
IWK Health Centre, Halifax, Nova Scotia, Canada

CHRISTINA RIGELSKY, MS, CGC
Genomic Medicine Institute, Cleveland Clinic, Cleveland, Ohio, USA

EMILY A. SCHONFELD, MD
Division of Gastroenterology, University of Colorado Anschutz Medical Campus, Aurora, Colorado, USA

BRAD T. TINKLE, MD, PhD
Division of Medical Genetics, Peyton Manning Children's Hospital, Indianapolis, Indiana, USA

DYSON T. WAKE, PharmD
Senior Clinical Specialist, Pharmacogenomics, Mark R. Neaman Center for Personalized Medicine, NorthShore University HealthSystem, Evanston, Illinois, USA

BROOKE WALLS, MD
Grube Family Fellow in Movement Disorders, Department of Neurology, Indiana University School of Medicine, Indianapolis, Indiana, USA

JOANNE WOJCIESZEK, MD
Associate Professor of Clinical Neurology, Indiana University School of Medicine, Indianapolis, Indiana, USA

Contents

> The collection of family history has always been a tool for genetic evalua-
> tion, but it remains an essential tool even in the age of genomic medicine.
> Patients may have a risk for a disease based on family history regardless of
> the results of genetic and genomic tests. How this information is collected
> is less important than that relevant information is collected in the first
> place. There are many tools for collecting medical and family history infor-
> mation both by hand and electronically. Genetic and genomic testing
> should always be interpreted in the context of the personal and family
> history.

> Historically, both pretest and posttest genetic counseling has been stan-
> dard of care for genetic testing. This model should be adapted for primary
> care providers (PCPs) willing to learn critical information about the test and
> key concepts that patients need to make an informed testing decision. It is
> helpful for PCPs to discuss a few initial patients with a genetic counselor to
> prepare for the key concepts of pretest and posttest counseling. This
> article provides guidance about the recommended level of involvement
> of PCPs based on the test indication, test complexity, disorder manage-
> ment, and the potential for psychosocial sequela.

> Pharmacogenomics (PGx) is a powerful tool that can predict increased
> risks of adverse effects and sub-therapeutic response to medications.
> This article establishes the core principles necessary for a primary care
> provider to meaningfully and prudently use PGx testing. Key topics include
> in which patients PGx testing should be considered, how PGx tests are or-
> dered, how the results are translated into clinical recommendations, and
> what further advancements are likely in the near future. This will provide
> clinicians with a foundational knowledge of PGx that can allow incorpora-
> tion of this tool into their practice or support further personal investigation.

most common autosomal dominant conditions of the nervous system. NF1 has a high degree of variability in clinical presentation, which may include multiple neoplasms as well as cutaneous, vascular, bony, and cognitive features. Some of these manifestations overlap with other genetic conditions. Accurate diagnosis of NF1 is important for individualizing clinical care and genetic counseling. This article summarizes the clinical features, diagnostic work-up, and management of NF1.

This article presents a nongeneticist's guide to understanding the genetics of Parkinson disease (PD), including clinical diagnostic criteria, differential diagnoses, symptom management, when to suspect a hereditary factor, a summary of autosomal dominant and recessive PD genes, and proposed algorithm for genetic testing. There is increasing availability of genetic testing for PD but there are few recommendations on how these tests should be used in clinical practice. This article guides clinicians on the overall management of patients with PD, with emphasis on determining which patients should have genetic testing and how to interpret the results.

Compared to clinicians previously surveyed, primary care providers employed in a health system known for clinical genomics were more likely to have ordered or referred a patient for genetic testing, but had only modestly more genetics training and reported similarly low levels of comfort answering patient questions about genetic risk. Most supported population genomic screening, reported willingness to get screened themselves, and judged a hypothetical patient's decision to be screened favorably relative to a similar patient's decision to decline screening. Stakeholder perceptions of the ethical appropriateness of nudging at-risk patients to discuss testing with counselors were mixed.

Foreword
A Long Road

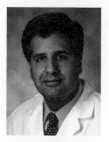

Bimal H. Ashar, MD, MBA, FACP
Consulting Editor

On June 20, 2000, President Bill Clinton delivered a speech describing the potential impact of the sequencing of the human genome: "We are here to celebrate the completion of the first survey of the entire human genome. Without a doubt, this is the most important, most wondrous map ever produced by human kind." President Clinton went on to say, "In coming years, doctors increasingly will be able to cure diseases like Alzheimer's, Parkinson's, diabetes and cancer by attacking their genetic roots."

Nearly 20 years after that speech, strides have definitely been made toward diagnosing and treating disease based on an individual's genetic makeup, especially cancer. However, we still have a long way to go. About 1 million people in the United States have Parkinson disease, while over 30 million people have diabetes, and 50 million people are afflicted by Alzheimer disease. The incidence of all of these diseases is increasing, with no imminent cures in sight.

In this issue of *Medical Clinics of North America*, Dr Howard Levy has assembled a team of experts to discuss where we are and where we are going with respect to genetic medicine. In addition to examining specific "genetic" disorders like neurofibromatosis and Ehlers-Danlos, the authors describe the potential impact of genetic medicine on more common disorders, the incidence of which was described above. Finally, the authors describe the potential impact of pharmacogenomics and whole-exome sequencing, topics of increasing importance to primary care providers, especially given the expansion of direct-to-consumer advertising.

The sequencing of the human genome was a remarkable achievement, one based in science and collaboration. Yet, much more needs to be done. As Chinese

Med Clin N Am 103 (2019) xv–xvi
https://doi.org/10.1016/j.mcna.2019.07.006
0025-7125/19/© 2019 Published by Elsevier Inc.

philosopher Lao Tzu said, "A journey of a thousand miles must begin with a single step." Sequencing was that first step.

Bimal H. Ashar, MD, MBA, FACP
Division of General Internal Medicine
Johns Hopkins University
School of Medicine
601 North Caroline street
#7143
Baltimore, MD 21287, USA

E-mail address:
Bashar1@jhmi.edu

Preface

Genetics for the Generalist: Yes, This Is Important for Your Patient

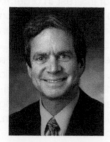

Howard P. Levy, MD, PhD
Editor

This issue of *Medical Clinics of North America* is about genetics. Unlike an organ system-focused or other specialty-based topic, the field of genetics truly touches on every specialty and every aspect of health and disease. There are hundreds of individually rare (but collectively common) single-gene Mendelian disorders, affecting every system, organ, tissue, and cell in the human body. But even more prevalent is the effect of multiple different genetic variants on predisposition to complex multifactorial diseases and the interaction between genetic variants and the environment. This includes not only what patients are exposed to in their day-to-day lives but also the various medications, radiation, and other factors we inflict upon them in an effort to diagnose, prevent, or treat disease. When considering this broadly, it is clear that genetics is too large topic for a single issue of any journal. Even selected highlights for the generalist will fail to adequately cover the field.

You will absolutely find authoritative and helpful information about many specific genetic conditions in the pages (or pixels) of this issue, and I encourage you to read each article herein. I also encourage you to look for common themes among and between these expert reviews.

Family history has always been the first, best, and least expensive genetic test. Obtaining, updating, and qualitatively interpreting the family medical history do not take much effort and can really help to inform your differential diagnosis, risk assessment, and preventive counseling. Even if there isn't a dominant, recessive, or x-linked condition in your patient's family, recognizing that the same or related disorders occur multiple times among family members will help you and your patient to identify the complex multifactorial conditions for which she or he is most at risk and possibly help you to disentangle the next confusing set of signs and symptoms she or he manifests.

Med Clin N Am 103 (2019) xvii–xviii
https://doi.org/10.1016/j.mcna.2019.07.005
0025-7125/19/© 2019 Published by Elsevier Inc.

Selecting, ordering and understanding genetic tests are also practical for generalists, once some basic principles are understood. Like all other tests, genetic tests are often clearly normal, sometimes clearly abnormal, and frequently somewhere in between. Variants of uncertain significance (VUS) are still quite common today. They will gradually become less common as we learn more about the genome, but for the next several years, it is important for all providers and patients to understand that a VUS is neither normal (benign) nor abnormal (pathogenic). If the differential diagnosis is very narrow, one should test only the one or few genes of interest in order to minimize the likelihood of finding a VUS that is unlikely related to the clinical question at hand. When the question is broader, sequencing of large panels of genes (or even the entire exome or genome) is reasonable but comes with more uncertainty.

Our genes do not define us and, with rare exception, the presence or absence of a pathogenic variant does not guarantee disease or lack thereof. Rather, our genetic makeup increases or decreases our risk of certain diseases (or, in the case of pharmacogenetics, of responding well to and tolerating a particular medication). Identifying disease-predisposing variants can help inform lifestyle modification for risk reduction, screening for earlier disease detection, and targeted therapeutic interventions.

If you've come here looking for information about a specific condition covered among these articles, I'm confident you'll find what you seek. I hope you'll also come away with more confidence incorporating the principles of genetics into your general or specialty practice.

Howard P. Levy, MD, PhD
Division of General Internal Medicine, Department of Medicine
McKusick-Nathans Institute of Genetic Medicine
Johns Hopkins University
Baltimore, MD 21205, USA

10753 Falls Road
Suite 325
Lutherville, MD 21093, USA

E-mail address:
hlevy3@jhmi.edu

Family Health History
The First Genetic Test in Precision Medicine

Robin L. Bennett, MS, CGC

KEYWORDS

- Family history • Medical family history • Pedigree • Pedigree nomenclature
- Donor gametes • Transgender

KEY POINTS

- Genetic and genomic testing should always be interpreted in the context of the patient's medical and family history.
- There are many methods of recording family history and there are a growing number of programs compatible with the electronic medical record.
- All health practitioners should know how to record a medical family history in the form of a pedigree, using standard pedigree nomenclature, and to provide a basic interpretation of this information.
- There are recommendations for pedigree symbols for complex personal and family relationships (eg, same-sex couples, pregnancies conceived with donor gametes, adoption, transgender, consanguinity).
- Simple red-flags of family history include a diagnosis at an earlier age than typical (50 years is a good age to remember for common adult-onset disorders), bilateral disease in paired organs, multifocal disease (eg, 2 primary cancers), and 2 or more closely related relatives on the same side of the family with the condition (especially if diagnosed at a young age).

INTRODUCTION

There are a plethora of genetic tests to consider in the evaluation and management of patients. A genetic test may be diagnostic, presymptomatic, or a screening test for healthy persons. Genetic tests are done on different tissues, such as blood or saliva (germline) or other tissues (somatic). These tests may be offered throughout the life-cycle: for pregnancy planning (preconception), prenatal (during a pregnancy), newborn screening, in childhood, and throughout adulthood. An underlying theme of all of these genetic tests and approaches is that genetic testing should always be interpreted in the context of the patient's medical and family history. A patient's medical family history is the first genetic test; it is a gateway for determining the approach

Disclosure: The author has nothing to disclose.
Division of Medical Genetics, Department of Medicine, University of Washington, University of Washington Medical Center, Box 357720, 1959 Northeast Pacific Street, Seattle, WA 98195-7720, USA
E-mail address: robinb@uw.edu

Med Clin N Am 103 (2019) 957–966
https://doi.org/10.1016/j.mcna.2019.06.002
0025-7125/19/© 2019 Elsevier Inc. All rights reserved.

medical.theclinics.com

to considering the need for genetic testing and the interpretation of the test results.[1–3] Family history can be provided by the patient in advance of the visit and confirmed by the practitioner or gathered at the clinic visit.

CORE INFORMATION TO INCLUDE IN MEDICAL FAMILY HISTORY

A medical family history is the compiling of key medical and demographic information about the patient and closely related biological relatives. Information is included about at least the first-degree relatives (children, full siblings, parents) and second-degree relatives (half-siblings, both sets of grandparents, and aunts and uncles). Third-degree relatives may also be included (first cousins, half-aunts and uncles). A 3-generation family history is considered minimum, but a more extensive family history may be required depending on the age of the person. For example, if a 40-year-old man is concerned about a family history of colon cancer in his sister and his paternal uncle, the history would likely include information about his children, siblings and their children (his nieces and nephews), his parents and their siblings (his aunts and uncles on both sides of the family), and his grandparents (at least on his father's side of the family). This approach compares with family history for an adolescent, which would likely be limited to health information about siblings, parents, aunts and uncles and their children, and grandparents (3 generations). Core health and demographic information to document for patients and their close relatives is noted in **Box 1**.

RED FLAGS OF MEDICAL FAMILY HISTORY

A major outcome from recording a patient's medical family history is to determine whether the clinician should be doing anything differently for this patient than usual and whether there are red flags in this family history that suggest the patient is at higher-than-average risk for a disease/disorder. Gathering this type of information does not need to be complicated. Early age of disease onset is one of the easiest

---

Box 1
Key health and demographic information to document in a family health history for the patient and closely related relatives

- Age (or year of birth)
- Age at death and cause of death (year if known)
- Siblings (distinguish whether half or full siblings)
- Children (note whether with separate partners)
- Miscarriages (particularly for a preconception or pregnancy consultation)
- Parents and grandparents
- Major health conditions, and the age at diagnosis (eg, cancer, aneurysm)
- Major surgeries (eg, cardiac, hysterectomy, oophorectomy, mastectomy, prostatectomy)
- Environmental exposures (eg, tobacco, alcohol, drugs)
- Occupational exposures (eg, asbestos exposure, mining)
- Country of ancestral origin for both sets of grandparents (if known)
- Whether a person's parents are closely related (first cousins or more closely related)

The date the information was collected, who provided the information, and who recorded the information should be noted.

alerts to remember to consider a hereditary condition; 50 years of age is a conservative cutoff for many common diseases (eg, cancer and heart disease). Another simple clue to think genetic is when 2 or more closely related relatives have the same condition on the same side of the family. A person who has more than 1 major health condition (eg, 2 primary cancers, hearing loss and retinal disease, 2 major vascular events, a seizure disorder and intellectual disability) may have a hereditary condition. A summary of the "signposts" in family history to think genetic are reviewed in **Box 2**.

ANCESTRY AND FAMILY HISTORY

Recording countries of origin for patients is important in genetic diagnosis and interpretation of genetic and genomic testing and should always be noted on a family history. Certain genetic disorders are more common in some populations because of founder mutations from a small pool of common ancestors. For example, there are 2 common pathogenic mutations in *BRCA1* (c.5266dupC and c.68_69delAG) and 1 in *BRCA2* (c. 5946delT) in the Ashkenazi population (Jews with ancestors from eastern Europe); thus 1 in 40 men and women of this ancestry is at risk to carry one of these pathogenic mutations. In Iceland there is a common pathogenic mutation in *BRCA2* (999del5) that is found in 0.6% of the population and is observed in 10.4% of women with breast cancer and 38% of men with breast cancers.[4] In Finland there is a spectrum of more than 30 mostly autosomal recessive disorders that occur more often in this population because of founder pathogenic mutations (http://findis.org/heritage. html, accessed March 13, 2019). Knowing the person's ancestry can help guide the approach to genetic testing. For example, a person who has a family history of breast or ovarian cancer might first be tested for the 3 common founder mutations seen in the Ashkenazi population before proceeding to full gene sequencing (which saves costs).

Knowing ancestry can also guide informed consent for genetic testing. However, most of the genetic population studies on normal and pathogenic variants for inherited disorders have been based on individuals of European ancestry. Therefore, individuals who are from underrepresented populations (eg, African, Asian, Latino, Native American, First Nation) have a higher likelihood of the identification of a genetic variant of uncertain significance than a person of European ancestry.[5] Although variants of uncertain significance (VUS) may be found in any person, patients from these populations should be forewarned of the higher likelihood of identification of a VUS in advance of any genetic testing. Likewise, the identification of carrier status for

---

Box 2
Signposts of medical and family history that suggest an inherited disorder

- Common disorders that occur at younger ages than typical
- A person with more than 1 major health condition or medical event
- Two or more relatives on the same side of the family with a health condition (particularly if earlier than typical age of onset)
- Bilateral disease in paired organs
- Two primary cancers (eg, breast and ovarian cancer, 2 primary colon cancers, prostate and colon cancer)
- Unusual presentation of the condition (eg, male breast cancer, lung cancer in a nonsmoker)
- Sudden death in a person who seemed healthy
- Medical problems in the offspring of parents who are consanguineous (first cousins or closer)

autosomal recessive disorders varies by ancestry (eg, the likelihood of identifying a common mutation in the cystic fibrosis gene, *CFTR*, is higher in persons of European ancestry than in persons of African ancestry).

OTHER IMPORTANT ELEMENTS

Individuals who are closely related (eg, first cousins) are at slightly increased risk to have children with a recessive disorder (because of inheriting a pathogenic mutation from a common ancestor).[6,7] Although the risk to develop a significant medical problem in the first years of life is low for the offspring of first cousins (a few percent higher than for nonconsanguineous couples), this information is important to note for genetic risk assessment, and a referral to genetic counseling may be important (particularly for couples who are pregnant or considering a pregnancy).

Age at time of diagnosis is also an important piece of information. For example, if a person has a first-degree relative with colon cancer at age 40 years, screening for colon cancer would be offered to the patient 10 years younger (age 30 years) even in light of that patient having a negative genetic test.

RECORDING A FAMILY HISTORY: A PEDIGREE IS A USEFUL TOOL

Any new patient to primary or specialty care should have key family history documented. Whether the collection method is through a standard paper table or checkbox that is scanned into the medical record, or through a graphical pedigree that is hand drawn or generated by a software program, the most important focus is to gather this information in the first place. There is a growing movement with the electronic medical record (EMR) and patient health portals to have patients generate the family history for the medical record and perhaps even to share this information electronically with their relatives. Welch and colleagues[8] summarize and review many of the electronic patient-facing family health history tools.

Recording a graphical family history in the form of a pedigree is a skill that all practitioners should be familiar with. The health information collected can be targeted by specialty (eg, cardiology, neurology, ophthalmology, oncology) or broader (eg, a first prenatal, pediatric, or primary care visit). With a pedigree, pages of health information can be compressed to 1 visual document through the association of simple symbols: squares, circles, diamonds, triangles, and lines. The square (male) or circle (female) can be shaded to track a condition (eg, aneurysm, cancer, seizures).

A pedigree has many advantages compared with a table format: the key health information can be tracked by the shading of the pedigree symbols so that patterns of inheritance can be more easily recognized. Autosomal dominant patterns showing transmission of disease from one generation to the next with both men and women affected are clearly visible. A preponderance of men affected in a pedigree might suggest an X-linked pattern of inheritance. If only 1 generation is affected, this may disclose autosomal recessive inheritance. If a person has family health information that does not identify conditions that run in the family, standard preventive health screening is likely the appropriate strategy.

Often the approach to genetic and genomic testing is to test the person who is most likely to have a positive test and then to provide cascade testing to other relatives, starting with first-degree relatives of the one who had a positive test. A pedigree is a visual tool to help determine who is the best person to test in the family and which other relatives should be tested.

All health professionals should be able to interpret the major symbols that are used to form a pedigree. Standard symbols for pedigree nomenclature, developed through a peer review process, are now considered the international standard, are included in major software pedigree drawing programs, and are being incorporated into the main EMR programs[9,10]; they are included in the American Medical Association Manual of Style, 10th Edition (http://www.amamanualofsyle.com/view/10.1093/jama/9780195176339.0, accessed March 13, 2019). Commonly used pedigree symbols are shown in **Figs. 1–3**.

When family history is recorded from a scanned health form or in simple text, often only positive health information is recorded. For example, the medical record may state "positive for grandmother and aunt with colon cancer." This information lacks important details, such as the age the relatives were diagnosed with cancer, whether they are living, or even whether they are on the same side of the family. In contrast, the clinician may report family history is negative or unremarkable. This information gives no clue as to the breadth of health information collected or the framework of the family structure. Is this information collected on a 50-year-old person and the person's 4 siblings, parents who are living in their 70s, and grandparents who died in their 90s, or is it on a 50-year-old person who is estranged from 1 or more parent and knows nothing about the extended family health history? A pedigree would provide the clinician with this information at a glance.

INCLUSIVE FAMILY HISTORY

Collecting family history is rarely straightforward. Blended families are common. It is important for genetic risk assessment to distinguish biological from nonbiological relatives (eg, step-siblings or a person who has been adopted). There may be misattributed paternity in a family that may not have been disclosed. A person may know little about a relative because of estrangement. A person may have been conceived by a donor gamete, or a surrogate may be involved with carrying a pregnancy. Gender identity may be nonconforming or a person may be transitioning gender. Many of these ways of representing relationships and identify are addressed in the National Society of Genetic Counselors 2008 recommendations.[1,10]

For individuals who are transgender, the gender identity can be used with the transition noted below the symbol (eg, male-transition-female would be a circle with MTF noted). A diamond can also be used for a person who is gender nonconforming or for a person who is transgender (and the transition noted as female to male, or male to female).

In all cases, it is important to be respectful of the person's identity and the family relationships.

THE FAMILY HISTORY INTERVIEW

When gathering information about a person's family history, whether in an electronic format or by a hand-drawn pedigree, it is useful to begin with the consultand (the person seeking medical attention), or the proband (the affected individual who brings the family to medical attention). An arrow is used to point out this person as a point of reference because the family history radiates out from this point to relatives by ascent (the parents, siblings, grandparents, and prior generations) and descent (the children and grandchildren). Adding names or initials can be helpful to keep track of who is who in the family. For healthy relatives who are related distantly, it is acceptable to record the number of relatives within a symbol (eg, a square labeled with a 3 would be 3 men, or a circle labeled with a 4 would represent 4 women).[10]

Asking open-ended questions is the best way to obtain a range of health information. A query of, "Describe the major medical problems that affect your parents" is

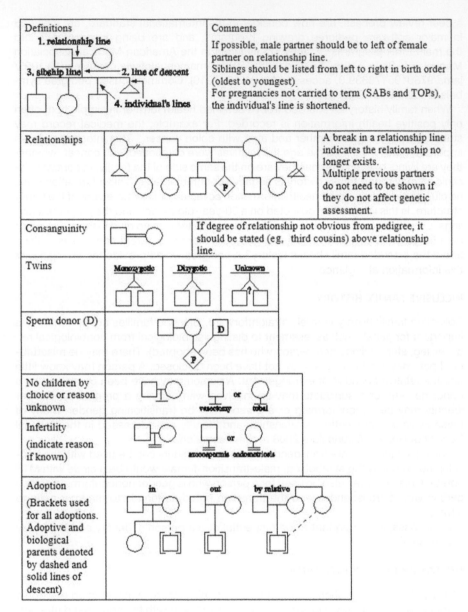

Fig. 1. Pedigree line definitions and common pedigree symbols. SAB, spontaneous abortion; TOP, termination of pregnancy. (*Adapted from* Bennett RL, French KS, Resta RG, et al. Standardized human pedigree nomenclature: update and assessment of the recommendations of the National Society of Genetic Counselors. J Genet Couns 2008;17(5):428; with permission.)

more likely to provide relevant information than "So, your parents are healthy?" It is helpful to have a systematic approach of asking questions starting with the patient, then extending to children (and grandchildren if appropriate), siblings, and then each parent and their siblings and parents. Specialty physicians ask questions in

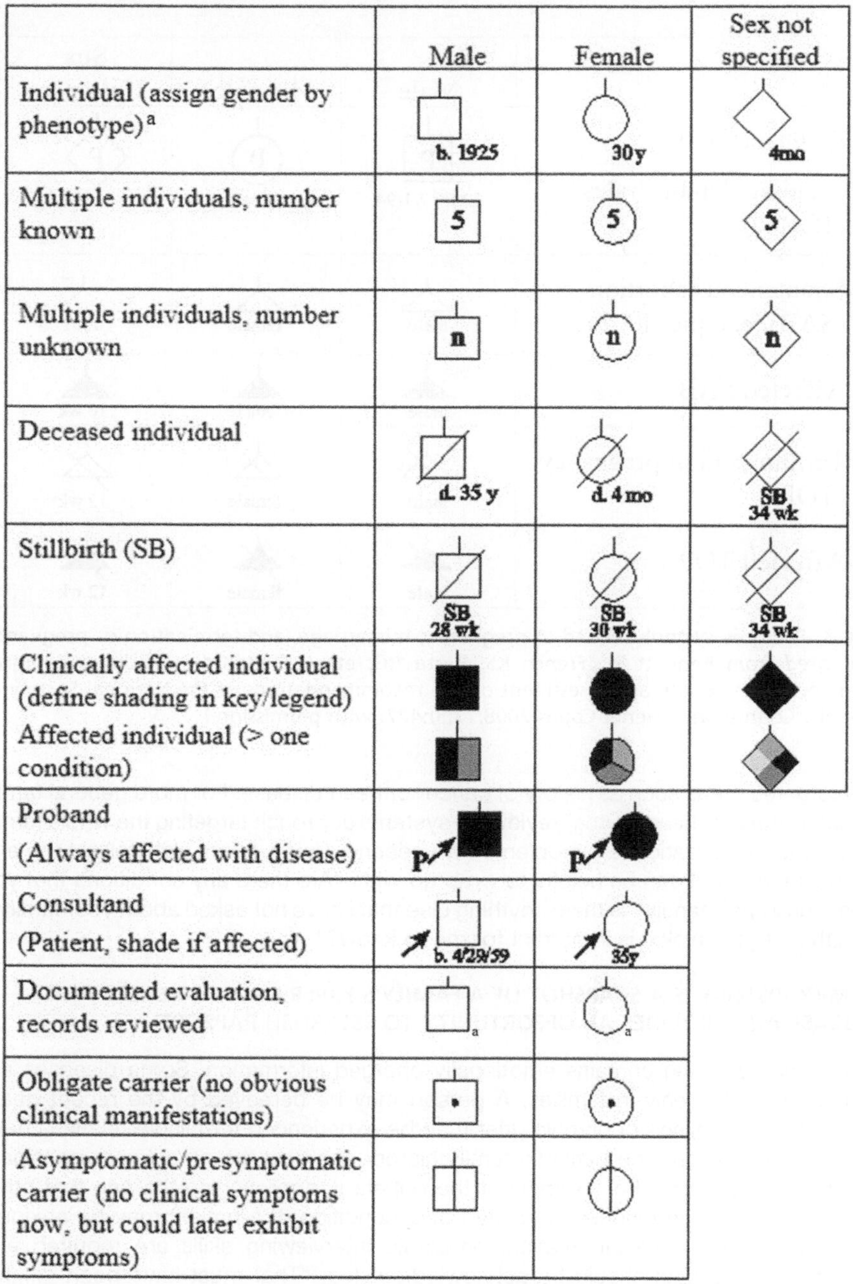

	Male	Female	Sex not specified
Individual (assign gender by phenotype)[a]	□ b. 1925	○ 30y	◇ 4mo
Multiple individuals, number known	5	5	5
Multiple individuals, number unknown	n	n	n
Deceased individual	◻ d. 35 y	⊘ d. 4 mo	◇ SB 34 wk
Stillbirth (SB)	◻ SB 28 wk	⊘ SB 30 wk	◇ SB 34 wk
Clinically affected individual (define shading in key/legend) Affected individual (> one condition)	■ ■	● ●	◆ ◆
Proband (Always affected with disease)	P↗ ■	P↗ ●	
Consultand (Patient, shade if affected)	↗ □ b. 4/29/59	↗ ○ 35y	
Documented evaluation, records reviewed	□a	○a	
Obligate carrier (no obvious clinical manifestations)	⊡	⊙	
Asymptomatic/presymptomatic carrier (no clinical symptoms now, but could later exhibit symptoms)	⊟	⊘	

Fig. 2. Additional pedigree symbols. [a] A diamond can be used for a person who is gender nonconforming and the sex at birth noted in text below the symbol. A diamond can also be used for a person who is transgender and the sex at birth noted or male-transition-female (MTF) or female-transition-male (FTM), as appropriate. The identifying gender symbol can also be used (eg, a square and FTM, or a circle and MTF). (*Adapted from* Bennett RL, French KS, Resta RG, et al. Standardized human pedigree nomenclature: update and assessment of the recommendations of the National Society of Genetic Counselors. J Genet Couns 2008;17(5):427; with permission.)

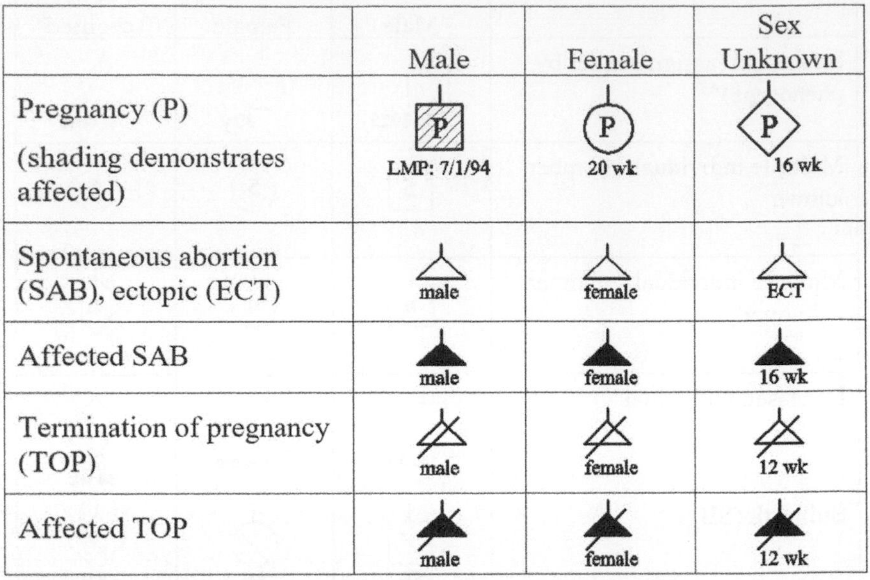

	Male	Female	Sex Unknown
Pregnancy (P) (shading demonstrates affected)	[P] LMP: 7/1/94	(P) 20 wk	<P> 16 wk
Spontaneous abortion (SAB), ectopic (ECT)	△ male	△ female	△ ECT
Affected SAB	▲ male	▲ female	▲ 16 wk
Termination of pregnancy (TOP)	⟋△ male	⟋△ female	⟋△ 12 wk
Affected TOP	⟋▲ male	⟋▲ female	⟋▲ 12 wk

Fig. 3. Pedigree symbols related to pregnancy, miscarriage, and termination of pregnancy. (*Adapted from* Bennett RL, French KS, Resta RG, et al. Standardized human pedigree nomenclature: update and assessment of the recommendations of the National Society of Genetic Counselors. J Genet Couns 2008;17(5):427; with permission.)

the targeted areas such as history of cancer or heart disease. For more general family health history, a "head-to-toe" review-of-systems approach targeting the whole family helps with organization (eg, problems with hearing, vision, heart, skeletal). At the end of the interview, it can be helpful to wrap up with, "Are there any conditions that you think run in your family? Is there anything else that I have not asked about your family's health that you think it is important for me to know?"[1]

FAMILY HISTORY IS A SNAPSHOT OF A FAMILY'S EXPERIENCE OF HEALTH AND DISEASE AND PROVIDES AN OPPORTUNITY TO ESTABLISH RAPPORT

Family history often contains emotionally charged information. Some diseases are not discussed openly in families. A person may be bereaved by the recent death of a relative. Feelings of chronic grief may be experienced if multiple relatives have died of a condition. The patient's family history can help the practitioner anticipate a patient's concerns. For example, if the patient is approaching the age that other relatives have been diagnosed or died of a condition, the patient may be anxious. As with any sensitive information, empathic interviewing skills are required and important life events should be acknowledged (eg, "That must have been difficult for you.").

Patients are more likely to comply with recommendations if they have a relationship with the clinician. Obtaining family health information is an excellent way to establish rapport with a patient. Patients are the experts on their family information, and this can be empowering for the patients. In this role as expert, the patients are more likely to be active participants in decisions about their health care. Patients are likely to feel listened to in the process of taking a family history, and this may even decrease patient anxiety.[1]

FAMILY HISTORY EVOLVES OVER TIME

When a medical family history is recorded, it is important to note the date the information was recorded and by whom; was this information recorded by the patient and reviewed by the practitioner or used from another clinic visit? Medical decision making is based on the information provided at that time; different decisions may be made with new information. Families change: relatives are born, die, and are diagnosed with diseases. Updates to family history (as new information is provided or at periodic visits) are important.

FAMILY HISTORY, GENETICS, GENOMICS, AND THE ELECTRONIC MEDICAL RECORD

The integration of family history information in the context of a patient's medical conditions and incorporation of genetic and genomic results is complex. An ideal state might seem to connect all relatives with a universal health record that would update as new information is known. For example, if someone's sister has a new diagnosis of breast cancer and has a pathogenic mutation in the BRCA1 gene, this information could be automatically uploaded into the person's file so that health providers would know what testing was needed. The practitioner may even receive an alert with clinical decision support, such as referral to a genetic counselor and/or for a genetic test.

Complications surrounding what may seem simple on the surface arise quickly. What about automatic disclosure of information that might be stigmatizing[11] (eg, mental illness, termination of pregnancy for a genetic indication, even a diagnosis of cancer that has not been shared with other relatives)? Can a person consent to sharing information with some relatives and not others? What about a child conceived by a donor sperm or donor egg; should the information about the health of the gamete donor be linked to that child's EMR and updated as health changes (for either the child or the gamete donor)? Should certain genetic information be specially protected (eg, presymptomatic test results for Huntington disease)? How is discrepant information dealt with in the EMR (eg, a man's pedigree says his father died at 50 years of age but his sister's pedigree notes he died at age 45 years; that age at diagnosis may denote different eligibility for genetic testing or recommendations for health screening).

SUMMARY

Family health history remains an essential tool in the application of genetic medicine. Even as genetic and genomic tools increase in availability, accuracy, and utility, the personal medical and family history continues to be the fulcrum on which interpretation of precision genomic medicine turns. The opportunities for family history in the electronic health history are vast, but the nuances of family structures and privacy must be seriously considered and respected. Medical and family history information can now potentially be collected and sorted from birth (or even prenatally) to grave. As more data accumulate on patients, their family histories, and concomitant genetic information, it is important that the critically important information for patient care be available in contrast with information overload. Dialogue between practitioners, specialists, genetics providers, software developers, laboratories, researchers, public health specialists, and patient advocacy organizations is necessary to continue to bring the power of medical family history and genomic health to fruition.

REFERENCES

1. Bennett RL. The practical guide to the genetic family history. 2nd edition. New York: Wiley Liss; 2010.

2. Pyeritz RE. The family history: the first genetic test, and still useful after all those years? Genet Med 2012;14:3–9.
3. Guttmacher AE, Collins FS, Carmona RH. The family history-more important than ever. N Engl J Med 2004;351:2333–6.
4. Tulinius H, Olafsdottir GH, Sigvaldason H, et al. The effect of a single BRCA2 mutation on cancer in Iceland. J Med Genet 2002;39:457–62.
5. Popely A, Fullerton SM. Genomics is failing on diversity. Nature 2016;538:161–4.
6. Bennett RL, Motulsky AG, Bittles AH, et al. Genetic counseling and screening of consanguineous couples and their offspring: recommendations of the National Society of Genetic Counselors. J Genet Couns 2002;11:97–119.
7. Hamamy HA, Antonarakis SE, Cavalli0Sforza LL, et al. Consanguineous marriages, pearls and perils: Geneva International Consanguinity Workshop Report. Genet Med 2011;13:998–1005.
8. Welch BM, Wiley K, Pflieger L, et al. Review and comparison of electronic patient-facing family health history tools. J Genet Couns 2018;27:381–91.
9. Bennett RL, Steinhaus KA, Uhrich SB, et al. Recommendations for standardized pedigree nomenclature. Am J Hum Genet 1995;56:745–52.
10. Bennett RL, French KS, Resta RG, et al. Standardized human pedigree nomenclature: update and assessment of the recommendations of the National Society of Genetic Counselors. J Genet Couns 2008;17:424–33.
11. Bennett RL. Pedigree parables. Clin Genet 2000;58:241–9.

Genetic Testing
Consent and Result Disclosure for Primary Care Providers

W. Andrew Faucett, MS, LGC[a],*, Holly Peay, MS, PhD, CGC[b],
Curtis R. Coughlin II, MS, MBe, CGC[c]

KEYWORDS

- Genetic testing • Informed consent • Genomic testing • ClinGen • CADRe
- Return of results

KEY POINTS

- Primary care providers (PCPs) can provide pretest consent for many genetic tests through a 15-minute to 30-minute targeted discussion or by a brief communication (discussion) and educational materials when management is straightforward.
- This model of PCPs providing pretest consent for straightforward testing situations improves access to genetic testing.
- Pretest and posttest genetic counseling by a licensed/certified genetic counselor should be considered for conditions with a high risk for adverse psychological impact or high residual risk.
- Genetic test result for a pathogenic variant (positive) may appropriately be disclosed by the ordering PCP along with referral to a genetic counselor.
- Genetic test result for a benign variant (negative) may often be disclosed by the ordering PCP with a targeted discussion or a brief discussion with educational materials.

INTRODUCTION

The use of genetic testing is growing in medical care, requiring primary care providers (PCPs) to play an expanding role in the consent and disclosure process. Historically many groups have recommended that both pretest and posttest genetic counseling be provided by a genetics-trained health care provider such as a genetic counselor

Disclosure: The work in this submission was funded by the NIH National Human Genome Institute 1U01HG007437.
[a] Office of the Chief Scientific Officer, Geisinger, MC 30-42, 100 North Academy Avenue, Danville, PA 17822, USA; [b] Center for Newborn Screening, Ethics, and Disability Studies, RTI International, 3040 East Institute Drive, Research Triangle Park, NC 27709, USA; [c] Department of Pediatrics, Section of Genetics, University of Colorado Anschutz Medical Campus, East 17th Avenue, Aurora, CO 80045, USA
* Corresponding author.
E-mail address: wafaucett@geisinger.edu
; @andyfaucett (W.A.F.)

Med Clin N Am 103 (2019) 967–976
https://doi.org/10.1016/j.mcna.2019.07.001
medical.theclinics.com

or medical geneticist, physicians who complete a medical genetics residency. Genetic counselors are masters level–trained allied health professionals who are certified by the American Board of Genetic Counseling and licensed in 26 states (www.nsgc. org, last accessed 8 February 2019). Although the number of licensed and/or certified genetic counselors (L/CGCs) continues to grow, there is only 1 genetic counselor or medical geneticist for every 132,000[1] and 650,000[2,3] persons in the United States respectively. There is a growing shortage of MD (Doctor of Medicine) clinical geneticists, and 46% of residency positions were unfilled in 2016. As the number of tests increases and clinicians become more familiar as testing moves into routine care, this model will limit access to testing, is not scalable, and most importantly this level of engagement with specialists may not be needed by many patients. The risk for psychological sequelae with most genetic testing has been shown to be low.[4] Many patients have an existing relationship with their PCPs, and access may be increased by not having to visit a different provider.

The CADRe (Consent and Disclosure of Recommendations) workgroup of the National Institutes of Health–funded Clinical Genome Resource (ClinGen) aims to increase access to genetic testing while maintaining effective communication and the patient-friendly experience historically provided by genetic counselors. To create a transparent process for determining appropriate provider/patient communication about genetic testing, we deliberated about situations in which consent and disclosure could be routinely managed by experienced PCPs; studied the issue through focus groups and surveys; and developed a rubric to categorize genetic tests and recommend the level of pretest and posttest genetic counseling based on test, disorder, and patient characteristics.[5] The output of CADRe work is used to justify the expanded role for PCPs in the pretest and posttest settings described in this article.

To prepare for the offer and disclosure of genetic testing, it is important that clinicians understand the benefits and limits of genetic testing and understand how to select appropriate tests for specific patients. Further, they must be comfortable with assessing patient understanding and comfort with genetic testing, returning what are sometimes complex results, making a genetic diagnosis, and knowing when to consult with or refer to genetics or other relevant specialties.

With the cost of testing decreasing, the ability to test for multiple genes in a single test, and growing online availability, the pretest work-up is less critical to choosing the patient-specific test. However, there will always be patients with an unusual presentation and/or unusual medical or family history who could benefit from consultation with a genetic counselor. PCPs should consider referring anxious patients or patients with the potential for psychological reactions to a genetic counselor. This article discusses the 3 levels of consent and disclosure interactions with patients and outlines the roles of the PCP and the genetic counselor.

As new tests enter the market it is important to work with individuals with genetic expertise (L/CGC) to adapt the recommendations in this article. Patients needing panel tests, exome sequencing, and genome sequencing may continue to benefit from consulting with an L/CGC.

CADRe's intention in developing the recommendations was that clinicians would start by considering CADRe's proposed level of communication, and then work with the patients to determine their preferred communication approach after taking into account the clinician's comfort and experience with the test and condition, the patient's baseline knowledge of the condition, and any underlying psychosocial concerns. Thus, this is intended to provide a baseline that is adjusted based on clinical judgment and preference.

Defining Levels of Communication

Three levels of patient communication at pretesting and posttesting were defined by CADRe and considered in their recommendations: traditional genetic counseling (ie, detailed discussion by an L/CGC), targeted discussion by an experienced and knowledgeable provider, and brief communication with educational and support materials. Those levels are described in **Fig. 1**. These levels were used to evaluate 2 stages of clinical interaction: pretest education and consent; and posttest disclosure, education, and support.

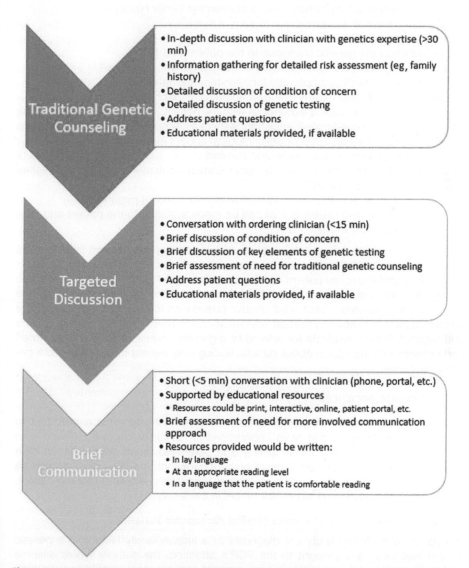

Traditional Genetic Counseling
- In-depth discussion with clinician with genetics expertise (>30 min)
- Information gathering for detailed risk assessment (eg, family history)
- Detailed discussion of condition of concern
- Detailed discussion of genetic testing
- Address patient questions
- Educational materials provided, if available

Targeted Discussion
- Conversation with ordering clinician (<15 min)
- Brief discussion of condition of concern
- Brief discussion of key elements of genetic testing
- Brief assessment of need for traditional genetic counseling
- Address patient questions
- Educational materials provided, if available

Brief Communication
- Short (<5 min) conversation with clinician (phone, portal, etc.)
- Supported by educational resources
  - Resources could be print, interactive, online, patient portal, etc.
- Brief assessment of need for more involved communication approach
- Resources provided would be written:
  - In lay language
  - At an appropriate reading level
  - In a language that the patient is comfortable reading

Fig. 1. Recommended communication strategies for genetic testing. Communication strategies differ regarding depth, and often length, of discussion. Key elements of each communication strategy are denoted as bullet points.

Factors that Affect Complexity of Pretesting and Posttesting Communication

CADRe identified a set of factors that influence clinical complexity, and thus drove recommendations about the appropriate degree of communication required for different patients:

1. Test complexity
   a. Is the choice of test to use obvious?
   b. Is the interpretation of the test result usually clear cut?
2. Testing situation complexity
   a. Is the patient symptomatic?
   b. Is the patient asymptomatic with a concerning family history?
   c. Is the patient at increased risk to carry a risk allele?
   d. Is the genetic cause in the family known?
3. Implication of the genetic diagnosis to the patient and family
   a. Is there guidance about management of the genetic condition?
   b. Is there no significant potential for near-term mortality?
4. Evidence of potential for adverse psychological impact
   a. Based on the clinician's experience with the patient, the patient's history, or the severity of the conditions in question, is there a low potential that the genetic test result will cause an adverse psychological impact in the patient?
5. Clinician knowledge, experience, and comfort
   a. Is the clinician comfortable managing pretest education and posttest results disclosure and support?
6. Availability of high-quality and patient-friendly educational materials
   a. Are there existing materials that can be made available to the patient and support the clinical interaction?

In general, when the answer to all of these questions is yes, referral to a genetics specialist (ie, an L/CGC) for pretest and/or posttest counseling is not always necessary. This model increases patient access and allows the PCP to manage the genetic testing. Additional details about how these test and patient-level variables should be factored into decisions about who should provide education and counseling are described later in relation to pretest education and consent and posttest disclosure and support. Patient requests for referral to a genetic counselor should be honored and patients with indecision about genetic testing may benefit from referral to a genetic counselor.

PRETEST COMMUNICATION

The education and testing consent process is an important step in the genetic testing sequence. Genetic tests can have implications for patients that are different than for many other types of clinical testing and screening, such as prediction of a later-onset disorder or exacerbation of presenting symptoms. Results may also be associated with treatment recommendations that may be unexpected for the patient, and results often have implications for others in the family.

Known Clinical Diagnosis or Known Familial Pathogenic Variant

If a patient already has a clinical diagnosis or a known family history of a genetic variant that they have brought to the PCP's attention, the authors would assume that a discussion of the condition's management and prognosis would occur during routine care and outside of the specific discussion of genetic testing. For these indications, we determined that a brief communication about genetic testing with the

PCP, together with the provision of educational resources, is sufficient for consent. The brief communication should ensure that the patient has sufficient knowledge about the condition, understands the risk based on the patient's relationship to the affected person in the family, appreciates what a positive and a negative genetic test result would mean, and wants to proceed with the testing. Supporting patient-friendly educational materials is important to ensure that the patient has additional resources as needed that can be accessed and reviewed as needed.

Clinical Symptoms Without Confirmed Diagnosis or Unknown Familial Variant

In situations in which a patient has a suggestive but not definitive clinical history, or if a patient is asymptomatic and at risk but with no causative variant identified in affected family members, the authors recommend a higher degree of communication: a targeted discussion with the ordering clinician about the condition and the potential outcomes of genetic testing. This discussion should include a more detailed discussion about the condition's natural history and prognosis; the importance of testing affected family members if possible; the testing process; the benefits and limitations of testing; implications for family members; the meaning of a positive, negative, or uncertain result; and anticipatory guidance about how the patient may feel on receiving all 3 types of results. The clinician should engage in shared decision making regarding the choice to be tested, including discussion of options if testing is declined.

Complex Testing or Significant Risk for Psychological Sequelae

Outside of these general recommendations, there are other major considerations for the degree of PCP communication and whether to refer to a clinical genetics specialist. Highly complex testing situations, such as complex testing with multiple possible causative genes, situations in which a negative result comes with a high residual risk of the condition, or unusual inheritance patterns should be referred to a genetics specialist. Conditions associated with an increased risk of an adverse psychological impact (eg, adult-onset progressive neurologic conditions and Huntington disease) benefit from referral to a genetics professional for pretest education and counseling. In addition, if the patient has a personal history or traits that lead the clinician to be concerned about a negative psychological response to the offer of and/or results from genetic testing, a referral to a genetic counselor (L/CGC) is warranted.

Significant Risk for Near-Term Mortality or Complex Management

For conditions with near-term risk of mortality or complex management, the authors recommend that, at minimum, PCPs undertake a targeted pretest discussion about the condition in question, the implications of both a positive and a negative test result for the patient and others in the family, and the patient's psychosocial readiness to receive the test results. Situations in which high-quality educational materials are not available to the patient also require clinicians to provide a higher degree of communication about the condition and/or test with the patient.

ALIGNING PRETEST COMMUNICATION WITH RESULTS DISCLOSURE

Depending on the test under discussion and the individual patient, communication of important information may occur in the pretest communication or the posttest communication. In general, most genetic test results can be returned to patients through a targeted or a brief discussion. Complex testing methods and genetic disorders associated with intricate management recommendations or significant psychological risk can complicate the disclosure process. Pretest genetic counseling by an

L/CGC in such cases is paramount. The detailed pretest discussion should include a plan for disclosure of testing results. As previously noted, pretest counseling for most patients consists of a targeted or a brief discussion. With this model it is likely that a disclosure plan is not formalized during the limited discussion, although discussion of a results disclosure plan is ideal. In cases in which a return of results plan has not been previously discussed, the type of genetic result can guide the PCP on the return of results process.

RESULTS DISCLOSURE

Genetic test results are far from binary. Although a positive (or pathogenic) result can confirm a clinical diagnosis, a pathogenic result may also be associated with a previously unknown disease risk. This risk can complicate the discussion because risk for disease is different from a diagnosis and can be difficult to understand for both patient and clinician. A crucial component of the results disclosure process ensures patients can understand the personal implications of the result. Whether a patient requires a detailed discussion or traditional genetic counseling about a result can depend on several factors, which include but are not limited to the implications of the result, the patient's personal or family history, and the patient's health and medical literacy. Furthermore, in genetics, positive and negative often have different meanings than other medical tests; a positive test can be positive for disease or risk and a negative test may mean that an answer was not found but the patient remains at risk. Genetic results (variants) may not always be associated with developing a disease. In order to aid the clinician, genetic variants are interpreted into one of the following categories: pathogenic, likely pathogenic, uncertain significance, likely benign, and benign.[6] In many cases, the category of the variant (ie, pathogenic or benign) can help guide the return of results process (**Table 1**).

Pathogenic and Likely Pathogenic Variants

The interpretation of genetic variants is based on the understanding of human biology, functional studies of the gene or protein, and population genetics.[6] Pathogenic and likely pathogenic results are highly associated with a disease phenotype. In the past, many health care providers referred to these results as positive, abnormal, or mutation found, which emphasized the degree of certainty associated with the results. A positive result for a risk allele (eg, *BRCA1* pathogenic variant) is not a diagnosis of disease and can require discussion to improve patient understanding.

Pathogenic and likely pathogenic results often have clear implications for the patient, and a targeted discussion by the patient's PCP is often appropriate for informed patients. There may be treatment guidelines or familial implications associated with a

Table 1
Method of genetic test result disclosure

Test Result	Method of Disclosure
Pathogenic or likely pathogenic variant	Targeted discussion (PCP) or L/CGC referral
Adult-onset conditions identified in a minor	L/CGC referral
Patient with a history of depression or anxiety	L/CGC referral
Variant of unknown significance	L/CGC referral
Benign or likely benign results	Brief discussion (PCP)
High residual risk caused by personal or family history	Targeted discussion (PCP)

pathogenic or likely pathogenic result. The disclosure process could include referral to an L/CGC or a targeted discussion about the result followed by a referral to a subspecialist for further management or a detailed discussion about the result and follow-up recommendations. The disclosure of a pathogenic or likely pathogenic result is similar to disclosure of most abnormal laboratory or imaging results familiar to PCPs. Discussion of a plan to share results with family members should be included. There are situations that may require a detailed discussion or a referral to a clinician with genetics expertise, which are detailed later.

Pathogenic Variants: Adult-Onset Conditions Identified in Minors

Decisions about whether to pursue genetic testing for adult-onset conditions in a minor are complex and should be focused on the best interest of the child.[7,8] As a result, a traditional genetic counseling model is recommended before pursing testing.[9] Occasionally, genetic testing is performed without pretest counseling or an adult-onset condition is an unexpected finding. In such situations, the result should be disclosed to the family or legal guardian.[10] The result disclosure process is complicated by several factors, including the need for a formal plan to disseminate the result to the patient at an appropriate age and possible psychosocial implications for the patient. As a result, disclosure of adult-onset conditions identified in a minor should include a detailed discussion (traditional genetic counseling) (L/CGC).

Pathogenic Variants: Patients with a History of Depression or Anxiety

Receiving a pathogenic genetic result can result in short-term depression and anxiety in any patient.[11] Significant depression or anxiety has been shown to be rare. The risk for depression or anxiety is complex and includes, but is not limited to, the nature of the genetic disorder and the patient's clinical status. Because of the increased risk of short-term stress, a detailed discussion or a referral to an L/CGC should be considered in patients with an existing history of anxiety or depression.

Variants of Unknown Significance

Variants of unknown significance (VOUS) are particularly difficult for PCPs and genetic specialists alike. These results are neither pathogenic nor benign, but a consequence of the current lack of knowledge, which results in a high degree of uncertainty. Not surprisingly, patients have reported feelings of anxiety, worry, and uncertainty when receiving VOUS.[12] Providing counseling may help relieve feelings of anxiety and uncertainty. In a survey of patients who received traditional genetic counseling, the risk perception of individuals with VOUS was similar to that of those who had a negative test.[13] Furthermore, the classification of VOUS is not static. Results are often reclassified in the future, which could affect medical decision making.[14] It is important to provide counseling focused on the uncertainty of the result and that the result may be reclassified to either a pathogenic or benign variant in the future. A plan for continual contact between the patient and provider should be established to address the possibility of variant reclassification. Traditional genetic counseling or a detailed discussion after the PCP consults with a genetics professional is recommended when a VOUS is identified.

Benign and Likely Benign Results

In almost all situations, a benign, likely benign, or no-variant-identified result should be treated as a negative genetic test result. Historically, many health care providers may have referred to a benign result as a polymorphism. By definition, a polymorphism is a genetic result that occurs at a frequency higher than 1% of the population. Pathogenic variants can be fairly common[15,16] and benign variants may be rare. With current nomenclature, benign indicates that the genetic result is not associated with a disease phenotype. As a result, most benign and likely benign results can be disclosed to patients through a brief discussion such as a phone call, an electronic patient portal, or through written material.

With no variant identified, the family and personal medical history can be important and referral for detailed discussion (genetic counseling) may be indicated. In genetics a negative only places the patient at population risk when a known familial variant is not found. Because of limitations of testing and knowledge, patients may remain at high risk after genetic testing when the familial mutation has not been identified (residual risk).

Disclosing genetic results using a brief discussion model has the same caveats as pretest counseling noted earlier. The decision to use written communication depends both on the patient and the ability to communicate key components about the benign result. It is important to communicate that both a benign and a negative result indicate that a genetic cause was not identified. This situation is not equivalent to stating that a patient does not have a genetic disease. A genetic cause may not have been identified because of the limitation of the testing (ie, incomplete or poor sensitivity testing), other genes not tested, or because of the limited understanding of the disease. In those patients with a clinical diagnosis of a genetic disease or patients in whom there is a high risk caused by a personal or family history, a targeted discussion about the benign results is warranted.

Results Disclosure and Further Considerations

Result disclosure is a process. It can begin with the PCP, and patients can be referred for genetic counseling or vice versa. The most important, and difficult, aspect of the results disclosure process is to identify what is in the best interest of the patient. The general guidelines discussed earlier depend on the patient, pretest counseling, and the clinician-patient relationship.

It may be evident to the PCP when a patient will benefit from genetic counseling or a patient may advocate for counseling following a result. Note that patients may desire genetic counseling, but may not request counseling, as a result of anxiety or worry over external judgment related to their need for further counseling.[17] As a result, all patients should be made aware that genetic counseling is available if needed or desired. The decision to refer a patient for genetic counseling should be patient centered, although there are situations in which genetic counseling should be strongly considered. In general, these situations mirror the need for genetic counseling before testing. Specifically, referral should be considered when a condition has a high risk for adverse psychological reactions or the testing is complex. Genetic counseling by an L/CGC may be necessary pretesting and posttesting or may only be necessary once during the testing process.

SUMMARY

PCPs are playing an increasing role in the provision of genetic testing by working with genetic counselors to understand the key points necessary for informed consent and the key points for results disclosure. PCPs can leverage their relationships with their patients to determine the level of pretest and posttest communication that will benefit the patient and increase access to genetic testing. There is a limited number of conditions for which testing is known to be associated with psychological reactions or choosing the best test can be complicated, and in these cases referral to a genetic counselor (L/CGC) is recommended. Working with a genetic counselor, there are many genetic tests with which PCPs can provide testing using targeted discussion or a brief discussion accompanied by educational materials and increase patient access to genetic testing.

CASE EXAMPLE

Listed here are examples to outline the interplay between pretest and posttest discussion.

BRCA1 and BRCA2 testing of a woman at increased risk caused by known familial mutation. Pretest consent was a brief discussion that did not include discussion of management. The patient has high medical literacy, already knows a lot about the condition based on family experience, and has no history of anxiety. Posttest discussion of a pathogenic variant should be a targeted discussion to include familial implications and management discussion. If the patient appears anxious, consider genetic counseling with L/CGC.

BRCA1 and BRCA2 testing of a woman at increased risk caused by family history and no family member with history of cancer available to test. Pretest consent was a targeted discussion that included limitations of testing because of lack of known pathogenic variant. Posttest discussion of pathogenic variant could be traditional genetic counseling (L/CGC) if the patient needs help with management of familial implications or a targeted discussion.

BRCA1 and BRCA2 testing of a woman at increased risk caused by known familial mutation. Pretest consent was a brief discussion that did not include discussion of management. The patient has high medical literacy and no history of anxiety. Posttest discussion of no mutation found (negative result) could be a brief discussion.

BRCA1 and BRCA2 testing of a woman at increased risk caused by family history and no family member with history of cancer available to test. Pretest consent was a targeted discussion that included limitations of testing caused by lack of known pathogenic variant. Posttest discussion of no mutation found (negative result) should be traditional genetic counseling or targeted discussion to consider additional testing and management decisions based on family history.

ACKNOWLEDGMENTS

This work was possible because of the work of members of the ClinGen CADRe workgroup: Kyle Brothers, MD, PhD; Adam H. Buchanan, MS, MPH, LCGC; Mildred Cho, PhD; Erin Currey; Miranda L.G. Hallquist, MSc, LCGC; Laura Hercher, MS, CGC; Louanne Hudgins, MD, FACMG; Seema Jamal, MSc, CGC, CCGC; Dave Kaufman, PhD; Howard Levy, MD, PhD; Nicole Lockhart, PhD; Kelly Ormond, MS, LCGC; Alice Popejoy, PhD; Erin Ramos, MPH, PhD; Myra Roche, MS, CGC; Maureen Smith, MS, CGC; Melissa Stosic, MS, CGC; Wendy Uhlmann, MS, CGC; and Karen Wain, MS, LCGC.

REFERENCES

1. National Society of Genetic Counselors: Genetic counselor workforce initiatives. Available at: http://www.nsgc.org/p/cm/ld/fid=532. Accessed October 5, 2017.

2. Summar ML, Watson MS. LDTs, incidental findings, and the need for more geneticists. Medscape 2015. Available at: http://www.medscape.com/viewarticle/853979. Accessed September 27, 2017.

3. Cooksey JA, Forte G, Flanagan PA, et al. The medical genetics workforce: an analysis of clinical geneticist subgroups. Genet Med 2006;8(10):603–14.
4. Ringwald J, Wochnowski C, Bosse K, et al. Psychological distress, anxiety, and depression of cancer-affected BRCA 1/2 mutation carriers: a systematic review. J Genet Couns 2016;25(5):880–91.
5. Ormond KE, Hallquist MLG, Buchanan AH, et al. Developing a conceptual, reproducible, rubric-based approach to consent and result disclosure for genetic testing by clinicians with minimal genetics background. Genet Med 2019;21(3): 727–35.
6. Richards S, Aziz N, Bale S, et al, ACMG Laboratory Quality Assurance Committee. Standards and guidelines for the interpretation of sequence variants: a joint consensus recommendation of the American College of Medical Genetics and Genomics and the Association for Molecular Pathology. Genet Med 2015;17(5): 405–24.
7. Committee on Bioethics, Committee on Genetics, and, American College of Medical Genetics and, Genomics Social, Ethical, Legal Issues Committee. Ethical and policy issues in genetic testing and screening of children. Pediatrics 2013;131(3): 620–2.
8. Ross LF, Ross LF, Saal HM, et al. Technical report: ethical and policy issues in genetic testing and screening of children. Genet Med 2013;15(3):234–45.
9. Botkin JR, Belmont JW, Berg JS, et al. Points to consider: ethical, legal, and psychosocial implications of genetic testing in children and adolescents. Am J Hum Genet 2015;97(1):6–21.
10. Green RC, Berg JS, Grody WW, et al. ACMG recommendations for reporting of incidental findings in clinical exome and genome sequencing. Genet Med 2013;15(7):565–74.
11. Mella S, Muzzatti B, Dolcetti R, et al. Emotional impact on the results of BRCA1 and BRCA2 genetic test: an observational retrospective study. Hered Cancer Clin Pract 2017;15:16.
12. Makhnoon S, Shirts BH, Bowen DJ. Patients' perspectives of variants of uncertain significance and strategies for uncertainty management. J Genet Couns 2019; 28(2):313–25.
13. Richter S, Haroun I, Graham TC, et al. Variants of unknown significance in BRCA testing: impact on risk perception, worry, prevention and counseling. Ann Oncol 2013;24(Suppl 8):viii69–74.
14. So M-K, Jeong T-D, Lim W, et al. Reinterpretation of BRCA1 and BRCA2 variants of uncertain significance in patients with hereditary breast/ovarian cancer using the ACMG/AMP 2015 guidelines. Breast Cancer 2019;26(4):510–9.
15. Burnham-Marusich AR, Ezeanolue CO, Obiefune MC, et al. Prevalence of sickle cell trait and reliability of self-reported status among expectant parents in Nigeria: implications for targeted newborn screening. Public Health Genomics 2016; 19(5):298–306.
16. Grosse SD, Gurrin LC, Bertalli NA, et al. Clinical penetrance in hereditary hemochromatosis: estimates of the cumulative incidence of severe liver disease among HFE C282Y homozygotes. Genet Med 2018;20(4):383–9.
17. Vos J, van Asperen CJ, Oosterwijk JC, et al. The counselees' self-reported request for psychological help in genetic counseling for hereditary breast/ovarian cancer: not only psychopathology matters. Psychooncology 2013;22(4):902–10.

Pharmacogenomics
Prescribing Precisely

Dyson T. Wake, PharmD[a], Nadim Ilbawi, MD[b],
Henry Mark Dunnenberger, PharmD[a], Peter J. Hulick, MD, MMSc[c],*

KEYWORDS

- Pharmacogenomic • Pharmacogenetic • Medication optimization
- Precision medicine • Adverse effects • Personalized medicine • Patient safety

KEY POINTS

- Pharmacogenomics (PGx) is the use of patient-specific genetic variations to guide medication selection.
- Genetic variations can cause changes in number or function of metabolic enzymes, drug receptors and transporters leading to increased risks of adverse effects or decreased therapeutic efficacy.
- With notable exceptions, PGx testing is best used to assess the risk of general suboptimal response rather than the potential for specific side effects or allergies.
- Guidelines exist to help clinicians understand how to use PGx results when they are available.
- PGx testing is a powerful tool but does not override the need for clinical assessment and judgment.

INTRODUCTION

The use of pharmacogenomics (PGx) and other genetic tools to guide medication selection and improve patient care is on the rise. The US Food and Drug Administration (FDA) currently provides information for 284 biomarkers in 214 medications, including multiple boxed warnings that recommend PGx testing before initiating therapy. Several companies are now marketing genetic testing directly to consumers.[1,2]

Disclosure Statement: P.J. Hulick, D.T. Wake and N. Ilbawi: None. H.M. Dunnenberger: Consultant for Admera Health and Veritas Genetics.
[a] Pharmacogenomics, Mark R. Neaman Center for Personalized Medicine, NorthShore University HealthSystem, 2650 Ridge Avenue, Evanston, IL 60201, USA; [b] Department of Family Medicine, NorthShore University HealthSystem, 6810 North McCormick Boulevard, Lincolnwood, IL 60712, USA; [c] Center for Medical Genetics, Mark R. Neaman Center for Personalized Medicine, NorthShore University HealthSystem, University of Chicago, Pritzker School of Medicine, 1000 Central Street Suite 610, Evanston, IL 60201, USA
* Corresponding author.
E-mail address: phulick@northshore.org

Med Clin N Am 103 (2019) 977–990
https://doi.org/10.1016/j.mcna.2019.07.002
0025-7125/19/© 2019 Elsevier Inc. All rights reserved.

However, education to providers on how best to incorporate these results, or whether a test is appropriate for their patient, has not kept pace with these new developments.[3,4]

Clinicians have noted interest in several potential benefits of PGx testing, including guidance on initiating new medications, mutually informed decision making, and a reduction of the "medication odyssey" to find a suitable regimen.[5] However, several studies have found that providers may have concerns about their ability to accurately interpret PGx results and optimally incorporate them into therapeutic decisions.[6] An important factor to consider is the time necessary to incorporate PGx counseling into the patient visit. Recent reviews of primary care providers' responsibilities have found difficulty with meeting the current preventative medicine recommendations alone in standard visit windows; let alone additional PGx concerns and questions.[7] However; it is also possible that through avoidance of adverse effects and optimization of patients' medication regimens, PGx guidance could *increase* the time available to providers and improve engagement with patients.

The goal of this article was to answer the most important questions a provider may have while first investigating PGx testing:

- Which patients are likely to receive benefits from PGx testing?
- How does one choose between PGx tests?
- How does a provider translate PGx results into meaningful clinical recommendations?
- Finally, what changes are anticipated in the PGx landscape in the coming years and how can providers stay abreast of this progress?

BACKGROUND

PGx is the understanding and extrapolation of variations in the patient's underlying DNA into therapeutic recommendations or more simply use of a patient's specific DNA variations to guide medication selection. Definitions for genetic terms can be found in **Table 1**. A variation occurs when one or more of the nucleotides are altered: switched, inserted, or deleted. The focus is on how such variation can cause alteration in metabolism or sensitivity to certain medications.

PGx variation is most typically captured by the "star" (*) system. A *1 is most often assigned to the default reference allele (haplotype) or wild-type/fully functional allele. When other haplotypes are present, other designations are assigned (eg, *2, *3). It is important to note that the *1 allele designation is often based on the subpopulation originally studied and may not represent the most common allele in every population. A laboratory will assign a *1 designation if no other variants are detected on their assay, thus a *1 designation does *not* preclude the possibility that other alleles affecting function are present. This is an important factor in deciding on a testing laboratory.

Somatic versus germline variation is an important distinction. Germline variations are found in DNA throughout the patient's body, including gamete cells, and can be inherited. Somatic variations occur in a specific body area and may spread further throughout the body through cell division, but are not present in gamete cells and cannot be inherited. PGx testing focuses on germline variations that exist within the patient since birth. One exception is the application of genomics-guided cancer treatment, which can be based on somatic changes in the tumor.

Another important dichotomy is reactive versus preemptive testing. Reactive testing is testing done in response to a clinical need. In contrast, preemptive PGx testing is completed before a specific need for the information.[8] The benefit of a preemptive

Table 1
Definitions of common terms

Term	Definition
Allele	One of 2 or more versions of a gene or single nucleotide polymorphism (SNP) at a given position on a chromosome.
Chromosome	A DNA structure composed of several genes.
Deoxyribonucleic acid (DNA)	A double helix structure created by patterns of 4 nucleotides: adenine (A), thymine (T), guanine (G), and cytosine (C).
Diplotype	Specific combination of 2 haplotypes. Each haplotype is of either maternal or paternal inheritance.
Gene	The DNA instructions for the formation of a protein.
Genome	An organism's entire genetic code.
Genotype	The patient's genetic code at the specific sites being assayed.
Haplotype	A specific combination of SNPs or variations in the DNA sequence occurring on the same chromosome
Phenotype	The expression of the patient's genetic code for a given gene. This can be defined at many levels, including enzymatic activity of the protein produced by a gene to a broader clinical implication, which might be a phenotype explained by the influence of multiple genes, as in warfarin metabolism.
Prodrug	A medication that is metabolized into a more active form after administration.
Single nucleotide polymorphism (SNP)	A variation or mutation in DNA that results in the change of one nucleotide for another or the addition or removal of a nucleotide

test is the avoidance of delay in utilizing the PGx test to guide therapy. With a shift toward preemptive testing, the focus for most providers will move to what should be done with genetic information rather than when it should be collected.

IN WHICH PATIENTS SHOULD A PROVIDER CONSIDER PGx TESTING?

PGx guidance is available in many areas of medicine, including psychiatry, cardiology, and pain management (**Table 2**).[9–13] Antidepressant medications represent a prime opportunity for the use of PGx as there are multiple equivalent therapeutic options. The American Psychiatric Association guideline for treatment of major depressive disorder (MDD) recommends that any of a dozen alternatives are all equally "correct" medications and it is left to patient and provider to eventually find the best option.[14] Many patients have inadequate response to their initial therapy and subsequent

Table 2
Commonly prescribed medications with pharmacogenomic guidance

Depression/Anxiety	Pain	Cardiovascular	Miscellaneous
• Selective serotonin reuptake inhibitors (SSRIs) • Tricyclic antidepressants (TCA) • Venlafaxine • Aripiprazole	• Codeine • Hydrocodone • Oxycodone • Tramadol	• Warfarin • Clopidogrel • Metoprolol • Carvedilol	• Proton pump inhibitors (PPIs) • Simvastatin • Phenytoin • Tacrolimus • Abacavir

These medications are described in pharmacogenomics (PGx) guidelines or have Food and Drug Administration labeling regarding a PGx interaction.

recommendations largely consist of choosing another "first-line" option. PGx clinical guidelines are available to inform the use of tricyclic antidepressants (TCAs) and selective serotonin reuptake inhibitors (SSRIs) based on CYP2D6 and CYP2C19 activity.[11,12] Recent studies have shown decreases in adverse effects and improvement in depression scores in patients who have PGx-guided antidepressant therapy.[15,16] Therefore, patients considering initiating a new antidepressant medication may benefit from the use of PGx testing.

PGx is especially enticing when considering the time span involved. SSRIs can take 4 to 6 weeks to demonstrate full therapeutic response.[17] The patient and provider could spend several months managing dose adjustments, appointments, and new prescriptions before determining that a single medication is ineffective. PGx testing could allow the provider to more rapidly determine if a lack of response represents an insufficient trial or belies an inherent issue with the medication.

The applicability of PGx testing depends in part on the potential severity of the reaction. Abacavir is used in the treatment of human immunodeficiency virus and has the potential to cause severe cutaneous adverse reactions (SCAR).[18] Although this risk is generally low, the HLA-B*57:01 variant is associated with a significantly increased risk of SCAR with abacavir. As a result, abacavir is not only contraindicated in those known to be positive for HLA-B*57:01, but FDA labeling recommends "All patients should be screened for the HLA-B*5701 allele prior to initiating therapy."[18]

Another area of extensive research is the use of PGx to guide the appropriate dosing of the anticoagulant warfarin. Beyond factors such as concomitant medications, other health conditions, and dietary vitamin K intake, genetic variations have been found to alter warfarin therapy.[19] Alterations in CYP2C9 can impair the metabolism of warfarin and changes in VKORC1 may increase a patient's sensitivity to warfarin therapy.[10,20]

PGx guidance based on these initial gene links led to interesting variability in the results of 2 major studies. The European Pharmacogenetics of Anticoagulant Therapy (EU-PACT) trial found PGx guidance was associated with greater time in therapeutic international normalized ratio range than standard dosing.[21] Concurrently the Clarification of Optimal Anticoagulation through Genetics (COAG) trial found PGx guidance did not improve warfarin control and in fact was associated with less effective management for black patients.[22] The juxtaposition of these results highlights the need to match PGx tests to the patient. Tests in these studies primarily interrogated for CYP2C9*2 and *3. Although these represent the most prominent loss of function alleles in White patients this is not the case for all populations. In Black patients, the most common loss of function allele is CYP2C9*8.[10] The EU-PACT trial was composed of more than 98% white patients, whereas more than 25% of those in the COAG study were black. Using a panel based on White genetic proportions to guide dosages of black patients led to more harm than benefit. Current guidelines recommend against the use of PGx guidance in patients of African ancestry if the assay covers only CYP2C9*2 and *3. The most recent guidelines incorporate CYP4F2 (which metabolizes vitamin K) and other variations relevant in specific patient populations.[10]

The use of codeine has recently been restricted to adult patients following new evidence for increased risks of adverse effects in the pediatric patient population. Case reports have demonstrated the potential for serious adverse reactions in infants of breastfeeding mothers who have consumed codeine.[23] A major component of these restrictions is that codeine is a prodrug and is activated into morphine largely by CYP2D6.[24] Genetic variations can significantly increase a patient's CYP2D6 enzymatic activity and cause a corresponding increase in the proportion of morphine leading to elevated risks for adverse effects. Similar reactions may be seen in other CYP2D6-mediated pain medications, such as tramadol, oxycodone, and hydrocodone.[13] PGx guidance has also demonstrated improvements in reduction of pain intensity for patients with reduced CYP2D6 enzyme activity.[25]

Several studies have demonstrated that a vast majority of patients have at least 1 clinically actionable variant that could affect prescribing. A 2014 study of more than 10,000 patients by Vanderbilt University found that 91% of patients had at least 1 clinically significant variation in the 5 genes tested.[26] Another group using a wider PGx panel found that more than 97% of patients had a least 1 variation linked to drug response and a median of 3 such variations.[27] Without a precise delineation of which patients should or should not receive testing, it is best to understand factors that may increase or decrease the potential value of PGx testing.

Studies have found patients are highly interested in PGx testing.[5,28] In particular, patients are interested in the opportunity to use PGx guidance in reducing side effects and guiding therapeutic selections.[29] Barriers to wider use also have been reported, such as concerns for cost or insurance reimbursement.[30] In addition, some surveys have indicated that patients are concerned with who may have access to the results.[31]

For all its benefits, PGx testing may not be right for every patient. Some questions or concerns cannot be answered by current PGx testing, and patients should be counseled to ensure that they are properly informed of what the tests can and cannot provide (**Table 3**).[27]

When evaluating whether PGx results should be used in a patient's care, there are 3 tenets that must be investigated:

1. The strength of literature supporting the interaction
2. The likelihood and severity of the clinical impact of the interaction
3. The risks associated with alternative therapies

PGx testing does not apply to every medication. Hundreds of medications have been investigated for links to genetic variants, but newer medications and those used by smaller patient populations may not have been examined yet. For other medications, there may exist only a small set of cases and studies focusing on narrow populations or with inconclusive results. Because of this lack of clarity, several organizations give a rating for the strength of evidence supporting a given PGx interaction.[32,33] The severity of the potential interaction may also sway the provider or patient's desire to incorporate PGx guidance.

In addition, providers must consider that any change in therapy is also associated with its own risks. If PGx guidance leads to the use of a second-line agent, providers should be cognizant that this could entail risk of therapeutic failure if the new agent is generally less effective or tolerated. Providers may also find themselves prescribing medications with which they have less familiarity or agents not covered by the patient's insurance.

Table 3	
What pharmacogenomics (PGx) can and cannot do	
PGx Can...	**PGx Cannot...**
• Identify medications with increased risk of adverse effects	• Predict all adverse reactions to medication
• Identify medications with increased risk of therapeutic failure	• Predict the risk of a *specific* side effect for all medication
• Help narrow therapeutic selection	• Determine the risk of future diagnosis with a disease or of sequalae
• Assist in predicting dosage for some medications	• Serve as a "magic bullet" that delivers a perfect regimen with no risks

Another important consideration is that PGx testing is not able to determine the "perfect" medication for the patient. A "clean" PGx result does not indicate that the medication will not cause side effects or that it will be therapeutically effective; it only means that no adverse PGx interaction was discovered. Such patients would still be expected to have the normal risk of side effects with treatment and the normal risk of therapeutic failure. Thus, PGx testing should be thought of more as a tool to reveal potential complications of therapy rather than to reveal the one best option for treatment.

HOW ARE PGx TESTS ORDERED?

PGx testing can be performed as either a single-gene assay or as a panel of dozens or more genes.[34] Early testing was primarily composed of assays of a handful of variants in a single gene, targeted at the most common and most impactful variants. Economies of scale and new technologies have allowed large increases in the number of genes and variations covered with nominal increases in cost. PGx testing via panels is becoming more common with companies now offering substantial panels at similar costs of a single gene test. Most PGx tests analyze a subset of variants (also called single nucleotide variants, or SNPs) known to be relevant for determining PGx haplotypes of clinical significance. This is in contrast to sequencing the entire gene to look for variations across the entire gene.

When determining which test or panel will best serve the patient or population, it is important to consider indications with therapeutic overlap. For instance, if testing is desired for *CYP2D6* and *CYP2C19* due to the possibility of initiating therapy with antidepressants, then it also may be prudent to consider whether PGx guidance for medications to treat cardiovascular and pain conditions will be of value to the patient.[10–12,35] A panel test may represent a nominal cost increase over the single-gene assay but deliver dividends by ensuring that commonly coprescribed medications are also reviewed.

PGx panels themselves are not homogeneous and can vary significantly in breadth and scope.[34,36] Most panels will cover several of the most well-studied and impactful genes. Panels can have different combinations of SNPs even for the well-studied, impactful genes, and this can contribute to why one laboratory may report a *1 designation versus a different laboratory that reports a more refined haplotype. Other genes may be included based on the creator's review of literature or expectation for future research. A panel purporting to have a large number of genes may not necessarily provide additional value to the patient, as not all variants provide equal clinical utility.

In fact, some variants can be incredibly rare outside of certain populations but may be fairly common within that group. For instance, the variant of HLA-B*15:02 that is associated with increased risk of SCAR in patients prescribed carbamazepine has an allele frequency of 0.04% in patients of European ancestry but a frequency of 6.88% in those of east Asian ancestry.[37] One panel may provide more value to a patient if it interrogates variations that are more closely in line with his or her ancestry.

It is also important to investigate what other alternative or special assays are provided by the panel. Multiple copies of the *CYP2D6* gene (such as duplications) occur in in approximately 1 in 8 patients and this number may be even larger in Black and Asian patients.[38] Duplication of the gene can cause increased enzymatic activity and may be clinically significant. However, not all panels can test for the presence or extent of gene duplications.

Beyond the contents of the panel are factors related to the ordering and use of the panel. Does it require a cheek-swab, saliva sample, or blood draw, and are any of these a potential issue for the patient? Will the results be available in a therapeutically necessary window? The manner in which the results are returned can differ drastically between laboratories. Some panels provide little beyond raw genetic data, some provide hard copies of interpreted PGx results and recommendations, and others are fully integrated into the electronic health record and allow for the use of sophisticated clinical decision support (CDS) tools.

Finally, it is also important to consider the potential cost of PGx testing. Patients have greatly varied means and desires to pay for PGx testing. Some are cost-insensitive and willing to pay substantial amounts upfront. For others, providers may need to be cognizant of which testing companies offer sliding scale pricing or other assistance.

HOW TO USE/INTERPRET PGx TESTING?

The goal of PGx testing is incorporation into your routine therapeutic decision process. One important aspect to remember about PGx testing, and indeed about any particular tool or test, is that it is only one piece of the larger patient picture. PGx testing should be used in conjunction with all other relevant factors, such as renal function, concomitant medications, and interacting disease states to determine the final risk-benefit analysis of treatment. A "normal" PGx result should not generally be used as justification to initiate a medication to which the patient previously experienced a severe adverse reaction just as a result indicating a patient may be at increased risk of therapeutic failure should not necessarily lead to cessation of currently effective therapy.

Depending on the gene and protein in question, different result structures and terminology may be used.[39] Some genes may be described in terms of the metabolic activity, some by their general function, and others as simply present or absent. Understanding why these descriptions are used is important in comprehending the underlying effect that the results represent.

The gene variants, called alleles, may be denoted using star allele nomenclature. Each star allele is denoted by an asterisk and then a number (eg, *1, *2, *17) and represents 1 or more SNPs that are inherited together. Star alleles are assigned activity levels, with *1 typically used to denote "wild-type" or the absence of any discovered variations. As this is a diagnosis of exclusion, the breadth of the panel may alter which patients are reported as *1.

Pairs of these star alleles, called diplotypes, are categorized into phenotypes describing their enzymatic activity; from poor to ultrarapid metabolism, as shown in **Table 4**. A normal metabolizer (NM), historically called an extensive metabolizer, typically has the expected or "average" amount of enzymatic activity and would be expected to have the normal chance of therapeutic failure and adverse events.[9,39] Intermediate (IM) and poor metabolizers (PM) have less enzymatic activity than the "average" patient; leading to increased exposure to the medication (or slower conversion of a prodrug to its active form). Conversely, rapid metabolizers (RMs) and ultra-rapid metabolizers (UMs) have increased activity.

Some gene results describe the general function of genes such as with SLCO1B1 (related to simvastatin), VKORC1 (related to warfarin), and OPRM1 (related to opioids).[39] Results for these genes may be reported as normal, intermediate, or poor function. Similar to the results of the metabolic enzymes, a normal function result indicates that the patient has the expected amount of function and typically does not require dose adjustment. Those described as intermediate or poor function have reduced functional activity, with poor representing the more profound loss of activity.

Table 4
Definition of phenotypes

Phenotype	Description	Effect on Medication Response
Ultrarapid Metabolizer (UM)	Significantly increased enzymatic activity	Medications metabolized by these enzymes would be expected to be eliminated at an increased rate. Affected medications would have reduced half-lives and have less time for the medication to fulfillits therapeutic objective. Patients would be at an increased risk of therapeutic failure due to the lower effective dose they would experience.
Rapid Metabolizer (RM)	Elevated enzyme activity but less than ultrarapid	Medications that are prodrugs activated by this enzyme would be expected to have a greater proportion of the active moiety. In this case, patients would be at increased risk of adverse effects due to the higher effective dose they would experience
Normal Metabolizer (NM)	The normal or expected amount of enzymatic activity	These patients are expected to have the normal or average amount expected risk of side effects and therapeutic response. In general, these patients do not require dose adjustment.
Intermediate Metabolizer (IM)	Decreased enzymatic activity	Medications metabolized by these enzymes would be expected to be eliminated at a decreased rate. Affected medications would have increased half-lives and remain active in the body longer, patients would be at increased risk of adverse effects due to the higher effective dose they would experience.
Poor Metabolizer (PM)	Minimal or absent enzymatic activity	Medications that are prodrugs activated by this enzyme would be expected to have a diminished proportion of the active moiety. In this case, patients would be at an increased risk of therapeutic failure due to the lower effective dose they would experience.

Results for genes such as human leukocyte antigens (HLA) may be described as "positive" or "negative."[39] HLAs are important pieces of immune function and patients with an actionable variant for one of these genes are at increased risk for severe adverse reactions with specific medications. Patients who are positive for HLA-B*58:01 are at an increased risk of hypersensitivity to allopurinol and those positive for HLA-B*15:02 are at increased risk for SCARs if treated with carbamazepine or oxcarbazepine.[40,41] For these genes, the proportional amount of activity provided by the gene is less important than the presence of the variant itself.

Beyond the terminology, the manner in which the results are presented or formatted can vary significantly between reports. Some are presented as raw genetic information and others as the final therapeutic recommendation. Reports may use proprietary iconography to describe the results with certain symbols indicating patients with expected increased risk of either side effects or therapeutic failure. Other reports may use a "traffic light" style representation with 3 main categories indicating medications expected to have normal risk (green), to be used with caution (yellow) or avoided (red). Results displayed in either format may cause a provider to oversimplify PGx results and ignore additional clinical considerations. A report may have any or all of these methods of conveying information and as each such system is different, care should be taken to fully understand the implications of each categorization.

PHARMACOGENOMIC RESOURCES

Because of the constantly shifting nature of genetic medicine, it is important to know how to stay apprised of further developments in the recommendations for testing or interpretation of results. Online resources have been created to ease this burden. The Clinical Pharmacogenetics Implementation Consortium (CPIC) and Dutch Pharmacogenomics Working Group provide guidelines with background evidence in support of their therapeutic recommendations.[9,33] The Genetic Testing Registry provides overviews regarding available genetic testing companies.[42] The Pharmacogenetic Knowledgebase (PharmGKB) provides a curated database of gene variations and their links to medications.[43] This may represent a good source for delving into upcoming or less known PGx interactions.

Primary literature may represent a great tool for specialists to stay abreast of relevant changes but may be too time-consuming for more general practitioners. There are several organizations (**Table 5**) that provide contact with programs using PGx and updates on the current state of evidence.[33,44] Collaboration or discussion with these groups can ensure that everyone is providing care at the highest level possible.

However, these resources may still require significant time to use and do not represent a sustainable solution for most providers. CDS systems are paramount for systemic adoption of PGx.[6,45] These tools can provide flags or alerts when a medication with potentially actionable PGx associations is ordered and direct the provider to either incorporate existing results into their decision process or facilitate the ordering of a PGx test.

CASE EXAMPLE

A 25-year-old woman who is in your clinic has a recent diagnosis of MDD and no other health concerns. She is currently taking no prescription medications and reports having "bad experiences with meds" in the past. She is hesitant to initiate an antidepressant medication but also reports that she has heard of genetic testing that can determine which medication she should use if she must begin one. She wishes to know more about this "DNA test."

Table 5
Brief descriptions of pharmacogenomics organizations

Organization	Abbreviation	Brief Description
Clinical Pharmacogenetics Implementation Consortium	CPIC	Creates clinical guidelines for the incorporation of PGx results into clinical decisions
Implementing GeNomics In pracTicE	IGNITE	Investigates and provides resources for the implementation of PGx into clinical practice
Electronic Medical Records and Genomics Network	eMERGE	Funded by the National Institutes of Health (NIH) to create and disperse information on the utilization of electronic health records to facilitate genetic medicine
Pharmacogenomics Knowledgebase	PharmGKB	NIH-funded repository of genetic variations and links to medications

PGx testing may decrease the trial and error necessary to find the correct medication and may alleviate some hesitancy from the patient to attempt pharmacotherapy. However, it is also important to counsel the patient on the current limitations of testing. Although the test may provide some delineation between suboptimal choices and those with the most promise, it is unlikely that the test will be able to highlight a single, best medication regimen. After counseling, she decides to proceed with PGx testing.

Several months later, the patient is ready to try pharmacotherapy. The results of the PGx test show that she is a CYP2D6 UM and a CYP2C19 IM. She wants to know what this means for her and which medications would be best. Her insurance will cover paroxetine, sertraline, or bupropion. After reviewing the CPIC and PharmGKB resources (see **Table 5**) you note paroxetine is metabolized by CYP2D6 and would be expected to have reduced efficacy in this patient, as it is eliminated more rapidly. Sertraline is metabolized by CYP2C19 and in patients with greatly reduced activity this can lead to increased rates of adverse effects. In general, CYP2C19 IMs retain sufficient enzymatic activity to process sertraline and current CPIC guidelines recommend initiating the normal starting dose of medication. Bupropion has no current PGx guideline recommendations.

You discuss these aspects with her and the general pros and cons of sertraline and bupropion. She indicates that her aunt takes sertraline and has not had any issues, Her aunt may have a different pharmacogenomic profile, so family history must be used cautiously. You decide to proceed with a trial of sertraline therapy at the normal starting dose.

The same patient, now 47, remains a loyal patient at your clinic. She has MDD for which she continues to take sertraline, as well as hypertension, hyperlipidemia, and atherosclerosis. She is scheduled to undergo percutaneous coronary intervention (PCI) in the next month and will be started on antiplatelet therapy. She calls and says that "The surgery doc says I have the wrong genes for the medication they were going to put me on" and wishes to understand more about the reaction. You discover that the team planned to initiate clopidogrel post PCI but received an alert based on her PGx test results.

Clopidogrel is a prodrug that is activated in the body primarily through CYP2C19. Patients with reduced CYP2C19 activity are at risk for reduced activation and thus reduced antiplatelet effect. CPIC guidelines recommend against the use of clopidogrel in CYP2C19 IM and PM. Prasugrel or ticagrelor are alternatives that do not demonstrate this reduced therapeutic efficacy. You discuss these elements with your patient and suggest that the surgery team consider the use of either antiplatelet alternative.

This is an example of the inherent benefits of preemptive testing. Although *CYP2C19* and clopidogrel have a demonstrated link, this PGx information may not be immediately available for many patients at the time of need and it may be detrimental to delay the procedure until PGx testing is performed. This patient was initially tested because of a concern regarding antidepressants. However, cardiovascular concerns are common in patients with MDD and those same genes also both provide guidance for cardiovascular medications, such as clopidogrel, metoprolol, and flecainide.[46] Other genes covered by her panel may assist with cholesterol medication selection, initiation of warfarin, or with selection of antipsychotic therapies if such comorbidities arise. PGx testing truly delivers life-long results that continue to benefit the patient's medication selection.

HOW MIGHT PGx TESTING CHANGE IN THE NEAR FUTURE?

One possible paradigm shift in the near future may be a greater use of next generation sequencing (NGS). Although current tests look for the presence of a few specific variants within a gene, NGS may return the patient's entire DNA sequence for the gene. This may allow for the detection of rare variations and better understanding of genetic function. But this deluge of new data also will create issues for researchers and clinicians, as there will be large quantities of "variants of unknown significance" without clear guidance. CDS also may need to be redesigned to allow the storage and use of the new structure of data.

The maintenance of existing CDS architectures and the formation of new programs for delivering data will represent a significant opportunity in the coming years. Several health systems have begun using CDS tools to integrate PGx data into the clinical decision process and provide information to providers at the time when it is most valuable. Such CDS tools will be paramount as PGx tests become more common and new formats for results and testing arise. Focus may also be applied to the development of patient-facing apps and portals through which the patient may interface with his or her providers and receive counseling on the results.

SUMMARY

As powerful as PGx may be, it is important to remember that it is just another tool that providers may use to improve their patients' care. It will not always be the best tool for the job and results should not override a provider's expertise. PGx itself is only one part of the larger paradigm shift that is personalized medicine.

In that same vein, providers should have a plan in place for what to do with results before the test is ordered. This is both to ensure that the clinical question being asked is one that PGx testing can answer and that the patient is able to receive the benefits of testing. It is not uncommon for the rationale for testing to be patient curiosity or general information gathering and such cases are reasonable as long as both the patient and provider properly understand the results returned.

The techniques of PGx testing and the manner in which results are dispersed will continue to evolve. CDS resources to store and interpret genetic medicine will become more prevalent and more powerful but the changes should focus on improving the integration of PGx testing into clinical workflows rather than just more sophisticated analysis for the sake of data.

Regardless of which laboratory results or data analysis tool is used, the end result always should be what is most beneficial to the patient. And as each patient is an individual with his or her own perspectives just as varied as the genetics described here, it is important to match the treatment to the patient's goals just as much as to the test results.

REFERENCES

1. Bloss CS, Schork NJ, Topol EJ. Direct-to-consumer pharmacogenomic testing is associated with increased physician utilisation. J Med Genet 2014; 51(2):83–9.
2. FDA. FDA authorizes first direct-to-consumer test for detecting genetic variants that may be associated with medication metabolism. 2018. Available at: https://www.fda.gov/NewsEvents/Newsroom/PressAnnouncements/ucm624753.htm. Accessed February 1, 2019.
3. Rohrer Vitek CR, Abul-Husn NS, Connolly JJ, et al. Healthcare provider education to support integration of pharmacogenomics in practice: the eMERGE Network experience. Pharmacogenomics 2017;18(10):1013–25.
4. Lemke AA, Hutten Selkirk CG, Glaser NS, et al. Primary care physician experiences with integrated pharmacogenomic testing in a community health system. Per Med 2017;14(5):389–400.
5. Lemke AA, Hulick PJ, Wake DT, et al. Patient perspectives following pharmacogenomics results disclosure in an integrated health system. Pharmacogenomics 2018;19(4):321–31.
6. Unertl KM, Field JR, Price L, et al. Clinician perspectives on using pharmacogenomics in clinical practice. Per Med 2015;12(4):339–47.
7. Yarnall KS, Pollak KI, Ostbye T, et al. Primary care: is there enough time for prevention? Am J Public Health 2003;93(4):635–41.
8. Weitzel KW, Cavallari LH, Lesko LJ. Preemptive panel-based pharmacogenetic testing: the time is now. Pharm Res 2017;34(8):1551–5.
9. Swen JJ, Nijenhuis M, de Boer A, et al. Pharmacogenetics: from bench to byte–an update of guidelines. Clin Pharmacol Ther 2011;89(5):662–73.
10. Johnson JA, Caudle KE, Gong L, et al. Clinical pharmacogenetics implementation consortium (cpic) guideline for pharmacogenetics-guided warfarin dosing: 2017 update. Clin Pharmacol Ther 2017;102(3):397–404.
11. Hicks JK, Bishop JR, Sangkuhl K, et al, Clinical Pharmacogenetics Implementation Consortium. Clinical Pharmacogenetics Implementation Consortium (CPIC) guideline for CYP2D6 and CYP2C19 genotypes and dosing of selective serotonin reuptake inhibitors. Clin Pharmacol Ther 2015;98(2):127–34.
12. Hicks JK, Sangkuhl K, Swen JJ, et al. Clinical pharmacogenetics implementation consortium guideline (CPIC) for CYP2D6 and CYP2C19 genotypes and dosing of tricyclic antidepressants: 2016 update. Clin Pharmacol Ther 2017;102(1):37–44.
13. Crews KR, Gaedigk A, Dunnenberger HM, et al. Clinical Pharmacogenetics Implementation Consortium guidelines for cytochrome P450 2D6 genotype and codeine therapy: 2014 update. Clin Pharmacol Ther 2014;95(4):376–82.
14. Practice guideline for the treatment of patients with major depressive disorder (revision). American Psychiatric Association. Am J Psychiatry 2000;157(4 Suppl):1–45.

15. Hall-Flavin DK, Winner JG, Allen JD, et al. Utility of integrated pharmacogenomic testing to support the treatment of major depressive disorder in a psychiatric outpatient setting. Pharmacogenet Genomics 2013;23(10):535–48.

16. Olson MC, Maciel A, Gariepy JF, et al. Clinical impact of pharmacogenetic-guided treatment for patients exhibiting neuropsychiatric disorders: a randomized controlled trial. Prim Care Companion CNS Disord 2017;19(2).

17. Frazer A, Benmansour S. Delayed pharmacological effects of antidepressants. Mol Psychiatry 2002;7(Suppl 1):S23–8.

18. ZIAGEN [Package Insert]. Research Triangle Park, NC: GlaxoSmithKline; 2015.

19. Cho SM, Lee KY, Choi JR, et al. Development and comparison of warfarin dosing algorithms in stroke patients. Yonsei Med J 2016;57(3):635–40.

20. Johnson JA, Gong L, Whirl-Carrillo M, et al. Clinical pharmacogenetics implementation consortium guidelines for CYP2C9 and VKORC1 genotypes and warfarin dosing. Clin Pharmacol Ther 2011;90(4):625–9.

21. Pirmohamed M, Burnside G, Eriksson N, et al. A randomized trial of genotype-guided dosing of warfarin. N Engl J Med 2013;369(24):2294–303.

22. Kimmel SE, French B, Kasner SE, et al. A pharmacogenetic versus a clinical algorithm for warfarin dosing. N Engl J Med 2013;369(24):2283–93.

23. Kelly LE, Rieder M, van den Anker J, et al. More codeine fatalities after tonsillectomy in North American children. Pediatrics 2012;129(5):e1343–7.

24. Thorn CF, Klein TE, Altman RB. Codeine and morphine pathway. Pharmacogenet Genomics 2009;19(7):556–8.

25. Smith DM, Weitzel KW, Elsey AR, et al. CYP2D6-guided opioid therapy improves pain control in CYP2D6 intermediate and poor metabolizers: a pragmatic clinical trial. Genet Med 2019. [Epub ahead of print].

26. Van Driest SL, Shi Y, Bowton EA, et al. Clinically actionable genotypes among 10,000 patients with preemptive pharmacogenomic testing. Clin Pharmacol Ther 2014;95(4):423–31.

27. Dunnenberger HM, Biszewski M, Bell GC, et al. Implementation of a multidisciplinary pharmacogenomics clinic in a community health system. Am J Health Syst Pharm 2016;73(23):1956–66.

28. Patel HN, Ursan ID, Zueger PM, et al. Stakeholder views on pharmacogenomic testing. Pharmacotherapy 2014;34(2):151–65.

29. Haga SB, Mills R, Moaddeb J, et al. Patient experiences with pharmacogenetic testing in a primary care setting. Pharmacogenomics 2016;17(15):1629–36.

30. Bielinski SJ, St Sauver JL, Olson JE, et al. Are patients willing to incur out-of-pocket costs for pharmacogenomic testing? Pharmacogenomics J 2016;17(1):1–3.

31. Haga SB, O'Daniel JM, Tindall GM, et al. Survey of US public attitudes toward pharmacogenetic testing. Pharmacogenomics J 2012;12(3):197–204.

32. Whirl-Carrillo M, McDonagh EM, Hebert JM, et al. Pharmacogenomics knowledge for personalized medicine. Clin Pharmacol Ther 2012;92(4):414–7.

33. Caudle KE, Klein TE, Hoffman JM, et al. Incorporation of pharmacogenomics into routine clinical practice: the Clinical Pharmacogenetics Implementation Consortium (CPIC) guideline development process. Curr Drug Metab 2014;15(2):209–17.

34. Vo TT, Bell GC, Owusu Obeng A, et al. Pharmacogenomics implementation: considerations for selecting a reference laboratory. Pharmacotherapy 2017;37(9):1014–22.

35. Scott SA, Sangkuhl K, Stein CM, et al. Clinical Pharmacogenetics Implementation Consortium guidelines for CYP2C19 genotype and clopidogrel therapy: 2013 update. Clin Pharmacol Ther 2013;94(3):317–23.
36. Bousman C, Maruf AA, Muller DJ. Towards the integration of pharmacogenetics in psychiatry: a minimum, evidence-based genetic testing panel. Curr Opin Psychiatry 2019;32(1):7–15.
37. Phillips EJ, Sukasem C, Whirl-Carrillo M, et al. Clinical Pharmacogenetics Implementation Consortium Guideline for HLA genotype and use of carbamazepine and oxcarbazepine: 2017 update. Clin Pharmacol Ther 2018;103(4):574–81.
38. Hosono N, Kato M, Kiyotani K, et al. CYP2D6 genotyping for functional-gene dosage analysis by allele copy number detection. Clin Chem 2009;55(8): 1546–54.
39. Caudle KE, Dunnenberger HM, Freimuth RR, et al. Standardizing terms for clinical pharmacogenetic test results: consensus terms from the Clinical Pharmacogenetics Implementation Consortium (CPIC). Genet Med 2017;19(2):215–23.
40. Hershfield MS, Callaghan JT, Tassaneeyakul W, et al. Clinical Pharmacogenetics Implementation Consortium guidelines for human leukocyte antigen-B genotype and allopurinol dosing. Clin Pharmacol Ther 2013;93(2):153–8.
41. Leckband SG, Kelsoe JR, Dunnenberger HM, et al. Clinical Pharmacogenetics Implementation Consortium guidelines for HLA-B genotype and carbamazepine dosing. Clin Pharmacol Ther 2013;94(3):324–8.
42. Rubinstein WS, Maglott DR, Lee JM, et al. The NIH genetic testing registry: a new, centralized database of genetic tests to enable access to comprehensive information and improve transparency. Nucleic Acids Res 2013;41(Database issue): D925–35.
43. Sangkuhl K, Berlin DS, Altman RB, et al. PharmGKB: understanding the effects of individual genetic variants. Drug Metab Rev 2008;40(4):539–51.
44. Volpi S, Bult CJ, Chisholm RL, et al. Research directions in the clinical implementation of pharmacogenomics: an overview of US programs and projects. Clin Pharmacol Ther 2018;103(5):778–86.
45. Hicks JK, Dunnenberger HM, Gumpper KF, et al. Integrating pharmacogenomics into electronic health records with clinical decision support. Am J Health Syst Pharm 2016;73(23):1967–76.
46. Fiedorowicz JG. Depression and cardiovascular disease: an update on how course of illness may influence risk. Curr Psychiatry Rep 2014;16(10):492.

Genetic Causes of Liver Disease
When to Suspect a Genetic Etiology, Initial Lab Testing, and the Basics of Management

Emily A. Schonfeld, MD[a], Robert S. Brown Jr, MD, MPH[b],*

KEYWORDS

- Genetic testing • Hemochromatosis • Gilbert syndrome
- Alpha-1 antitrypsin deficiency • Wilson disease
- Progressive familial intrahepatic cholestasis
- Benign recurrent intrahepatic cholestasis • Lysosomal acid lipase deficiency

KEY POINTS

- The most common cause of hereditary hemochromatosis is a C282Y mutation in the HFE gene with a penetrance of 10% to 52%.
- Gilbert syndrome is a common and benign cause of indirect hyperbilirubinemia with no signs of hemolysis and no associated liver injury.
- Alpha-1 antitrypsin deficiency causes both lung and liver disease.
- Wilson disease can cause neurologic disease and liver disease.
- Progressive familial intrahepatic cholestasis is a rare cause of chronic cholestasis in children and young adults. Benign recurrent intrahepatic cholestasis is a benign cause of recurrent cholestasis seen in both adults and children.

INTRODUCTION

When evaluating a patient with liver disease, investigating genetic causes of liver disease is an important part of the workup. The initial evaluation of a patient with liver disease includes a history and physical examination. Obtaining a thorough family history plays a critical role because it can help determine which patients to consider for

Disclosures: The authors have nothing to disclose.
This is an update of an article that first appeared in the *Clinics in Liver Disease*, Volume 21, Issue 4, November 2017.
[a] Division of Gastroenterology, University of Colorado Anschutz Medical Campus, 1635 Aurora Court, 7th Floor, Aurora, CO 80045, USA; [b] Division of Gastroenterology and Hepatology, Weill Cornell Medical College, 1305 York Avenue, 4th Floor, New York, NY 10021, USA
* Corresponding author.
E-mail address: rsb2005@med.cornell.edu

Med Clin N Am 103 (2019) 991–1003
https://doi.org/10.1016/j.mcna.2019.07.003
medical.theclinics.com

genetic testing. However, a negative family history does not rule out genetic causes of liver disease. The age of onset of liver disease and the pattern of abnormal liver function tests (LFTs), hepatocellular or cholestatic, play a role in what testing is performed. This article reviews common genetic causes of liver disease, when to suspect a genetic cause of liver disease, laboratory testing required for diagnosis, and general management practices. Usually if there is a high suspicion of an inherited liver disease, it is important to refer to a specialist for diagnostic testing and management.

HEREDITARY HEMOCHROMATOSIS

Most (80%–90%) cases of hereditary hemochromatosis are caused by an autosomal recessive mutation in the *HFE* gene; specifically, the most common genetic mutation is homozygosity for C282Y.[1–7] Two less common mutations are H63D and S65C, which usually only cause signs and symptoms of iron overload when present as compound heterozygotes with C282Y.[1,3,8] Hemochromatosis secondary to the *HFE* gene mutation occurs from the unrestricted transfer of iron from the intestine into the blood leading to toxic levels depositing in various organs, including the liver.[9] Among patients with any type of liver disease, 3% to 5.3% are homozygous for C282Y, and therefore, an evaluation for hemochromatosis should be performed in the workup of liver disease of unknown cause or in patients with iron overload on laboratory testing or liver imaging.[4,8] Patients with hereditary hemochromatosis can present with other symptoms owing to iron overload, such as chondrocalcinosis, diabetes mellitus, heart failure, or porphyria cutanea tarda.[1,4,5,9,10]

HFE-associated hereditary hemochromatosis is most commonly seen in Caucasians of Northern European descent.[1,5,8] About 6% to 10% of Caucasians have 1 allele for C282Y and 0.3% to 0.5% have 2 alleles.[3,4,9] Of patients homozygous for C282Y, 10% to 52% develop clinical signs of iron overload.[1,4–9,11] Manifestations of hereditary hemochromatosis are more prevalent in men and present earlier in men, likely in part because of menstruation and therefore iron loss in women.[1,4,5,7,12]

The initial screening tests for hereditary hemochromatosis include blood tests for ferritin and transferrin saturation, which is calculated from iron/total iron binding capacity.[1,4] Transferrin saturation greater than 45% should prompt genetic testing for *HFE* gene mutations.[1,3–5,8,9] *HFE* gene testing usually tests for specific mutations, C282Y, H63D, and S65C. An increased ferritin level is expected in hereditary hemochromatosis, but is not highly specific; thus, an increased ferritin level with normal transferrin saturation is not common in hereditary hemochromatosis and should lead to investigation into alternative causes of liver disease.[9,13] Testing for advanced fibrosis or cirrhosis should be performed in patients who are homozygous for C282Y or compound heterozygotes for C282Y who have a ferritin level greater than 1000 μg/L, hepatomegaly, age more than 40 years, or abnormal liver tests.[1,4,5,12,14] A liver biopsy is not always necessary because MRI can evaluate for cirrhotic morphology and can quantify the amount of iron in the liver, and transient elastography can also be used to evaluate for advanced fibrosis.[4,15,16] The decision of whether to perform imaging tests versus a liver biopsy to evaluate for advanced fibrosis should be referred to a specialist.

In patients with laboratory testing consistent with iron overload, but who are not C282Y homozygotes, other causes of liver disease should be considered.[1,9,15] Whether C282Y heterozygotes or H63D homozygotes develop liver disease without other coexistent causes remains controversial. Iron overload is common in other liver diseases, such as alcohol-related liver disease, nonalcoholic fatty liver disease (NAFLD), and viral hepatitides.[1,9,13,15,17] In this situation, a liver biopsy may be necessary to investigate for alternative causes of liver disease.[1] Liver biopsies should be stained with Perls' Prussian blue to determine the amount of iron and the location of iron present.[1,15] Iron overload can be seen in cirrhosis of any cause; however, in hemochromatosis, the distinguishing feature is that iron is deposited in the fibrous septa, bile ducts, and walls of the vasculature as well as hepatocytes.[15]

If hepatic iron overload is suggested by laboratory testing, imaging, or biopsy, but workup for HFE genes and other causes of liver disease is negative, non-HFE genetic hemochromatosis should be suspected and secondary iron overload (eg, hemolysis) should be ruled out.[4,9,15] Less common genetic causes of hereditary hemochromatosis include juvenile hemochromatosis, mutations in transferrin receptor-2, mutations in ferroportin, aceruloplasminemia, atransferrinemia, and African iron overload.[1,18] Given the rarity of these mutations, a referral to a specialist for genetic testing should be made.[4,9,15]

Phlebotomy is the main treatment used for HFE-associated hemochromatosis and should be started when the ferritin is above normal.[1,4,9,19,20] Phlebotomy frequency is based on targeting a ferritin of 50 to 100 μg/L while trying to avoid causing anemia.[1,4] Food and supplement recommendations for patients with hemochromatosis include limiting or avoiding supplementation with vitamin C because this can increase mobilization of iron and avoiding raw shellfish because there is a described increased risk of infection with Vibrio vulnificus.[1,4,20] Limiting alcohol intake in patients with any type of liver disease is also a good recommendation.[4] If hemochromatosis patients do develop cirrhosis, they will need ongoing monitoring for hepatocellular carcinoma (HCC) with imaging every 6 months, similar to patients with cirrhosis from any cause.[4]

When a patient is identified as having HFE-associated hereditary hemochromatosis, it is important to screen their siblings for this disease.[1,4,7] Both parents of an affected patient are usually carriers of a mutation in the HFE gene, although they could be asymptomatic homozygotes because of incomplete penetrance. At diagnosis, about 4.4% to 11.8% of C282Y homozygous male patients have cirrhosis and 0% to 2.7% of C282Y homozygous female patients have cirrhosis.[6,9,12] Therefore, early diagnosis is important because initiation of phlebotomy before the development of cirrhosis can reduce or stop the progression of liver disease and eliminate the risk of HCC and improve survival.[1,12,19] Not all complications of hereditary hemochromatosis can be reversed with phlebotomy, such as arthritis and hypogonadism.[4,9] Phlebotomy can improve diabetes control, and even in patients with cirrhosis, may improve portal hypertension.[1,19,20] Iron can deposit in the heart as well as other organs and lead to arrhythmias and a cardiomyopathy, although this is less common in HFE forms of hemochromatosis and more common in juvenile hemochromatosis.[1,4,9]

Disease	Common Laboratory Abnormalities	Presentation of Disease
Hereditary hemochromatosis (HFE form)	↑AST/ALT Transferrin saturation >45% ↑Ferritin Gene testing, most commonly C282Y homozygote	Abnormal LFTs Cirrhosis HCC Diabetes mellitus Heart failure Hypogonadism Arthritis
What test to order? HFE gene mutation testing		

Abbreviations: ALT, alanine transaminase; AST, aspartate transaminase.

GILBERT SYNDROME

Gilbert syndrome is a benign cause of unconjugated hyperbilirubinemia in people with no liver disease or hemolysis.[21] It is caused by reduced bilirubin glucuronidation, a process needed to excrete bilirubin. The prevalence is about 1.6% to 10% of the population.[21–23] The bilirubin levels can fluctuate, but are usually between 1 and 5 mg/dL, always with a normal direct (conjugated) bilirubin level.[21,22,24,25] In adults, it does not lead to clinically significant liver disease.[21,23] Patients have normal aminotransferase and alkaline phosphatase levels, and their hemolysis workup is negative with no other physical examination findings to suggest liver disease.[21,24] In studies that have evaluated liver biopsies in these patients, normal histology was noted, and a liver biopsy is not needed for diagnosis.[24] Thus, patients with isolated unconjugated hyperbilirubinemia and no other evidence of liver disease should be reassured and require no further workup. Gilbert syndrome is more prevalent in men than in women, and fasting can increase the serum bilirubin level.[21,23]

Disease	Common Laboratory Abnormalities	Presentation of Disease
Gilbert syndrome	+ Unconjugated bilirubin	Fasting increases bilirubin level

ALPHA-1 ANTITRYPSIN DEFICIENCY

Alpha-1 antitrypsin is a protease inhibitor (Pi) produced in the liver that works to inhibit neutrophil elastase, which degrades proteins.[26–29] Alpha-1 antitrypsin deficiency is an autosomal recessive disease that can lead to panacinar emphysema as well as liver disease.[26,28,29] In contrast, emphysema in patients without alpha-1 antitrypsin deficiency is usually located in the lung apex.[26] Smoking in alpha-1 antitrypsin deficiency can lead to early-onset emphysema.[26] Alpha-1 antitrypsin deficiency should be suspected in patients with these manifestations or other rarer manifestations, such as panniculitis, often at sites of trauma, and vasculitis, which is usually c-ANCA (cytoplasmic antineutrophil cytoplasmic antibody) positive.[29–31]

There are multiple variants of the alpha-1 antitrypsin genotype, and some of these variants produce normal levels of alpha-1 antitrypsin, whereas some lead to reduced levels.[28] The reduced levels are associated with disease.[28] The null phenotype leads to no production of alpha-1 antitrypsin.[28] The normal alpha-1 antitrypsin phenotype is labeled MM, and severe deficiency is ZZ.[26,32,33] The ZZ phenotype most commonly leads to liver disease.[26,32,33] Less commonly, the SZ phenotype and the M_{malton} phenotype can lead to liver disease.[28,34] The prevalence of alpha-1 antitrypsin deficiency is about 0.02% to 0.06% in Caucasians, and heterozygosity for the MZ phenotype occurs in about 2% to 3% of Caucasians.[26,27,29,32,35]

Adult patients with alpha-1 antitrypsin deficiency can present with abnormal liver tests, usually elevated transaminases or bilirubin, and/or cirrhosis.[26–28,35,36] Alpha-1 antitrypsin deficiency is a more common cause of liver disease in men than in women.[34–36] In patients with alpha-1 antitrypsin deficiency and cirrhosis, patients should be followed for HCC.[33]

Patients with abnormal LFTs should be evaluated for alpha-1 antitrypsin deficiency, especially if they have a family history of liver disease or emphysema in a non-smoker. The screening examination evaluates the level of alpha-1 antitrypsin in the blood, and when low levels are found, further testing for abnormal phenotypes or genotypes is performed.[26,29,32] For patients with a first-degree relative with alpha-

1 antitrypsin deficiency, one can proceed directly to phenotype and genotype testing.[26,29,32] Some experts do phenotyping at the time of initial evaluation. Normal alpha-1 antitrypsin protein (referred to as M) and some abnormal proteins (eg, S and Z) can be diagnosed via Pi isoelectric focusing of the protein, but some abnormal proteins and complete absence of protein cannot be diagnosed by this method.[26,29,32] Patients with normal isoelectric focusing but low alpha-1 antitrypsin level require evaluation of the alpha-1 antitrypsin gene (SERPINA1) for a pathogenic mutation.[26,29,32]

Alpha-1 antitrypsin is an acute phase reactant, and levels can be increased in the presence of high estrogen levels, which can cause a false-negative test.[26,29,37] Low alpha-1 antitrypsin levels can also be seen in diseases associated with protein loss, such as via the kidneys or gastrointestinal tract.[26] A liver biopsy may be necessary to rule out other causes of liver disease. When a liver biopsy is performed, the alpha-1 antitrypsin enzyme is retained in hepatocytes and appears as periodic acid-Schiff positive, diastase-resistant globules in hepatocytes.[26,27,37]

Intravenous augmentation therapy, which is pooled purified human plasma alpha-1 antitrypsin, is used for the treatment of alpha-1 antitrypsin deficiency associated lung disease and can be used for panniculitis, but it does not improve the liver disease.[26,29] There is no therapy for the liver disease associated with alpha-1 antitrypsin deficiency other than liver transplant, and the transplant cures the deficiency.[28,38]

Disease	Common Laboratory Abnormalities	Presentation of Disease
Alpha-1 antitrypsin deficiency	+ AST/ALT + Alkaline phosphatase Phenotype analysis, most commonly ZZ	Early emphysema, especially in smokers Cirrhosis HCC

What test to order?
  Alpha-1 antitrypsin level; if low, then
  Alpha-1 antitrypsin isoelectric focusing; if normal, then
  SERPINA1 genetic testing		

WILSON DISEASE

Wilson disease is caused by an autosomal recessive mutation in ATP7B, which helps transport copper into bile and bind copper to ceruloplasmin.[18,39–42] The incidence is as high as 0.003%.[18,41–44] The mutation in ATP7B leads to copper deposition in the liver as well as the brain, kidneys, and cornea leading to varying manifestations of the disease.[18,41]

Wilson disease most commonly presents between 5 and 40 years old, but it should be considered in patients of any age with liver abnormalities, especially if a patient has symptoms suggestive of Wilson disease.[41] Patients with Wilson disease can present with no symptoms, a mild increase in aminotransferase levels, hepatomegaly, neurologic symptoms, or acute liver failure with a Coombs-negative hemolytic anemia and acute kidney injury.[41,44–46] Many patients already have cirrhosis at presentation, which is usually present by the second decade of life.[40,41,45,46] A small percentage of patients present with hemolysis alone.[41,44]

Neurologic changes seen in Wilson disease usually present in the third decade of life, but small changes in childhood, such as handwriting or behavior, can be seen.[40,41,43] The neurologic findings in Wilson disease are usually parkinsonian characteristics, such as rigidity and dystonia, as well as dysarthria, and brain imaging can detect abnormalities in the basal ganglia, although this is not diagnostic.[41,43] Patients may also present with psychiatric disorders.[41,43] Patients with neurologic symptoms from Wilson disease are often cirrhotic at the time of diagnosis.[43,47]

Ceruloplasmin can be used as an initial screening examination for Wilson disease, and a level less than 20 mg/dL leads to further testing.[48] However, Wilson disease cannot be completely ruled out if patients have normal ceruloplasmin, but other clinical symptoms are suggestive of the disease.[48,49] Kayser-Fleischer rings, caused by copper deposition in the cornea and diagnosed by slit-lamp eye examinations, are seen in 44% to 62% of patients with hepatic Wilson disease and in about 85.5% to 95% of patients with neurologic Wilson disease.[40,41,43,50] Kayser-Fleischer rings are not specific for Wilson disease because they can be seen in patients with chronic cholestasis from other forms of liver disease.[43,50] Ceruloplasmin is also an acute phase reactant, and its levels can be increased in patients with elevated estrogen, for example, during pregnancy.[41,43–45,48,50] Ceruloplasmin levels can also be low in patients who are losing proteins via the kidneys or gastrointestinal tract, in end-stage liver disease, or with aceruloplasminemia.[41,43,44] Therefore, if a ceruloplasmin level is normal, but there is still a high suspicion for Wilson disease, a 24-hour urine copper test can aid in diagnosis.[43,48]

If a low ceruloplasmin level (<20 mg/dL), high 24-hour urine copper level (>40 µg), and Kayser-Fleischer rings are present, then the diagnosis of Wilson disease is confirmed.[40,41,47,48,51] If only 2 of the 3 tests are positive, then a liver biopsy for histology and quantification of copper level (>250 µg/g dry weight of liver) are necessary and can help rule out other causes of liver disease.[40,41,43,44,49] Copper quantification of a liver biopsy can be important to help diagnose Wilson's disease because a liver biopsy in patient's with Wilson's disease can appear similar to biopsies from patients with NAFLD and can show signs of cholestasis, which does not distinguish it from other types of liver disease.[40,41,43,52] Copper staining of the liver biopsy is not useful because it is variable in patients with Wilson disease.[49] Genetic testing can be performed if patients have an intermediate hepatic copper quantification (50–250 µg/g) or if they have an increased urine copper level and Kayser-Fleischer rings, but do not meet the cutoff for copper quantification in the liver.[41,43,47] In addition, an increased free serum copper level (not bound to ceruloplasmin) may aid in the diagnosis, although it can be increased in other causes of acute liver failure, cholestatic liver disease, and in a copper overdose.[40,43–45]

In patients who present with acute liver failure caused by Wilson disease, classic findings include Coombs-negative hemolytic anemia, acute kidney injury, increased serum aminotransferase levels less than 2000 IU/L, and a normal or low alkaline phosphatase test.[41,43–45] Patients who present with acute liver failure usually already have cirrhosis at presentation.[43] The diagnosis of acute Wilson disease is critical because it does not respond to chelation or any medical therapy, and thus, urgent liver transplant is indicated and the only effective therapy.

Those patients with a first-degree relative with Wilson disease should be tested for the disease.[40,41,43] Genetic testing can be used as the primary means of diagnosis if the affected relative's genotype is known, because there are multiple mutations on ATP7B that have been identified, and patients can be compound heterozygotes.[40,41,43,44]

Once the diagnosis of Wilson disease has been made, treatment involves using the chelating medications, D-penicillamine or trientine, or zinc.[40,41,43,53] Both D-penicillamine and trientine can lead to worsening of neurologic Wilson disease when first

Disease	Common Laboratory Abnormalities	Presentation of Disease
Wilson disease	+ AST/ALT Low or normal alkaline phosphatase level Low ceruloplasmin level +24-h urine copper + Serum-free copper + Hemolysis workup Genetic analysis with *ATP7B* mutation	Hepatomegaly Cirrhosis Neurologic symptoms Acute liver failure Kayser-Fleischer rings
What test to order? Ceruloplasmin; if low, then 24-h urine copper; if high, then Evaluation for Kayser-Fleischer rings and/or Consider a biopsy with hepatic copper quantification If workup positive or concerning for Wilson disease, can then send *ATP7B* genotype		

started.[40,41,43] Liver transplant cures the underlying Wilson disease.[41,43] A low copper diet is also recommended, which means avoiding such foods as shellfish, nuts, chocolate, mushrooms, and organ meats.[41]

PROGRESSIVE FAMILIAL INTRAHEPATIC CHOLESTASIS

Progressive familial intrahepatic cholestasis (PFIC) encompasses 3 autosomal recessive mutations that lead to chronic cholestasis: PFIC1, PFIC2, and PFIC3.[54] PFIC is a rare disorder, and it is the cause of liver disease in about 10% to 15% of children with cholestatic liver tests.[54–58] Patients with PFIC can present with jaundice, pruritus, splenomegaly, and hepatomegaly.[54,55,59] Specifically, patients with PFIC1 and PFIC2 usually present at a few months of age, whereas patients with PFIC3 usually present later in childhood or early adulthood and usually present with cirrhosis.[54,55,59] Despite cholestatic abnormalities on their liver tests, patients with PFIC1 and PFIC2 have normal gamma-glutamyltransferase (GGT) levels, whereas patients with PFIC3 have increased GGT levels.[54,55,59] All 3 classifications of PFIC have increased serum bile acid levels.[54,55,59]

LFTs, GGT, and imaging studies help to rule out other more common causes of liver disease before diagnosing PFIC.[54,55,57] A liver biopsy may aid in the diagnosis of PFIC, and genetic testing can confirm the diagnosis of PFIC, although in a small number of patients the genetic defect may not be elucidated because some genes likely remain unidentified.[54,56,60] Family history is important in the evaluation of PFIC because cases of heterozygous mutations for the PFIC proteins have been found in women who developed intrahepatic cholestasis of pregnancy.[54]

Treatment is geared toward the normalization of LFTs and pruritis symptoms, and patients are usually started on ursodeoxycholic acid (UDCA). A biliary diversion can be performed if there is no or only partial improvement in pruritis to UDCA and other medications used to treat pruritis.[61,62] When patients have progressive liver disease, they may eventually need a liver transplant.[61,62]

Disease	Common Laboratory Abnormalities	Presentation of Disease
PFIC3	+ Alkaline phosphatase + ALT + GGT	Jaundice Pruritus Splenomegaly Cirrhosis in late childhood and young adulthood
What test to order? *ABCB4* gene testing		

BENIGN RECURRENT INTRAHEPATIC CHOLESTASIS

Benign recurrent intrahepatic cholestasis (BRIC) is an autosomal recessive disease caused by a mutation in the same genes as in PFIC; however, BRIC is a benign disease.[54] BRIC is a rare disease that can present in both childhood and adulthood and leads to recurrent episodes of cholestasis.[62] Each episode of cholestasis can last for a variable amount of time, and the time between episodes can range from weeks to years.[63,64] Between episodes, the patients are asymptomatic with normal liver tests.[63,64] During the recurrent episodes of cholestasis, patients with BRIC develop jaundice, pruritus, increased serum bile acid levels, increased alkaline phosphatase levels, a conjugated hyperbilirubinemia, and a low GGT level.[62,63] BRIC, unlike PFIC, does not progress to chronic cholestasis or cirrhosis.[62]

If a liver biopsy is performed during an episode of cholestasis, it shows cholestasis but no signs of chronic liver disease.[54,62,63] In order to diagnose BRIC, the patient must have at least 2 episodes of cholestasis with a symptom-free interval, and alternative causes of cholestasis must be excluded, which usually includes imaging, laboratory tests, and likely a liver biopsy.[63] The diagnosis can be supported by genetic testing, which would show a mutation in the same genes that are mutated in PFIC.[54,63]

Treatment is aimed at alleviating pruritis symptoms, and a liver transplant has been done for this.[62]

Disease	Common Laboratory Abnormalities	Presentation of Disease
BRIC	During episodes of cholestasis: + alkaline phosphatase + Conjugated hyperbilirubinemia + Serum bile acids Normal GGT Between episodes of cholestasis: Liver tests normal	During episode of cholestasis: jaundice Pruritus

LYSOSOMAL ACID LIPASE DEFICIENCY

Lysosomal acid lipase deficiency (LAL-D) is a rare autosomal recessive disorder that leads to problems with cholesterol metabolism.[65] It is a lysosomal storage disorder caused by a lack of, or deficiency in, liposomal acid lipase, which ultimately leads to accumulation of cholesterol in different organs and macrophages.[61,63,65,66]

LAL-D has different variations. The most severe form of LAL-D is called Wolman disease, which presents in early childhood, usually at 2 to 4 months of age.[65–68] Cholesteryl ester storage disease (CESD) is a different form of LAL-D that can present later in childhood or in adulthood and cause hepatosplenomegaly, dyslipidemia, accelerated atherosclerosis, and liver disease.[65,66] The different LAL-D phenotypes are based on the level of activity of lysosomal acid lipase.[66] Patients with Wolman disease have either no functioning enzyme or less than 1% activity, which is in contrast with CESD, which has a higher level of activity and therefore later onset.[66]

CESD is most common in Caucasians of European descent.[65,66] It is due to a mutation in the *LIPA* gene.[69] In North America, the prevalence of CESD is about 0.0008% in Caucasian and Hispanic populations.[69]

When evaluating cholesterol levels, these patients have high triglyceride and total cholesterol levels with low high-density lipoprotein (HDL) levels.[65,66,70] After being ruled out for other more common causes of liver disease, a liver biopsy in these patients can show microvesicular steatosis and birefringent cholesterol ester crystals or their remnant crystals in hepatocytes as well as lipids in the Kupffer cells.[65,66,68,71,72] The liver biopsy can be mistaken for NAFLD or cryptogenic cirrhosis, which can make it harder to diagnose adults with the disease.[65,66] A dried blood spot aids in diagnosis because it helps determine the peripheral leukocyte LAL activity, and a low activity would support the diagnosis of LAL-D.[65,66,68,71,72] Genotype analysis is not necessary for diagnosis, but a mutation in *LIPA*, the gene for LAL, is diagnostic.[65,66,70]

Patients have variable results to lipid-lowering agents in improving cholesterol.[65,66] Enzyme replacement therapy is available, which has improved survival in infants and improved transaminases in children and adults with this disease.[65] Patients may ultimately need a liver transplant if they have progressive underlying liver disease.[65,66]

Disease	Common Laboratory Abnormalities	Presentation of Disease
LAL-D	+ AST/ALT + Alkaline phosphatase Decreased peripheral leukocyte LAL activity in blood CESD: + Triglycerides + Total cholesterol, low HDL level	Hepatomegaly Splenomegaly
What test to order? *LIPA* genotype		

SUMMARY

In the genetic causes of liver disease described in this article, screening tests are used to suggest the diagnosis before sending genetic testing. Not all of the genetic diseases described have complete penetrance, and therefore, genetic testing may not be diagnostic. It is also important to evaluate for and rule out other more common causes of liver disease before genetic testing is performed. It is reasonable to go straight to genetic testing in patients who have a first-degree relative with a genetic cause of liver disease, especially if early intervention can prevent progressive disease.

Genetic causes of liver disease lead to a wide range of presentations, from mildly abnormal liver tests to acute liver failure. This article describes hereditary hemochromatosis, Gilbert syndrome, alpha-1 antitrypsin deficiency, Wilson disease, PFIC, BRIC, and LAL-D.

The most common cause of hereditary hemochromatosis is a mutation in the C282Y gene. If this genotype is absent, it is important to rule out other causes of liver disease because alcohol-related liver disease, NAFLD, viral hepatitis, and all causes of cirrhosis can present with blood tests consistent with iron overload.

Gilbert syndrome is a benign cause of indirect hyperbilirubinemia with no signs of hemolysis.

The phenotype that commonly causes liver disease in alpha-1 antitrypsin deficiency is PiZZ. Patients can present with increased aminotransferase levels, jaundice, cirrhosis, or emphysema.

Wilson disease can cause both neurologic disease and liver disease. Patients can present with a spectrum of liver disease from increased aminotransferase levels to fulminant liver failure.

PFIC can cause chronic cholestasis, and patients usually present between the neonatal period and young adulthood. It is a rare disorder, and other causes of cholestasis should be excluded first.

BRIC is a benign cause of recurrent cholestasis that does not lead to chronic liver disease. Patients with BRIC have a normal GGT level during the episodes of cholestasis.

Patients with CESD demonstrate microvesicular steatosis and cholesterol accumulation on liver biopsy and therefore can be difficult to distinguish from patients with NAFLD.

REFERENCES

1. Bacon BR, Adams PC, Kowdley KV, et al. Diagnosis and management of hemochromatosis: 2011 practice guideline by the American Association for the Study of Liver Diseases. Hepatology 2011;54(1):328–43.
2. Cheng R, Barton JC, Morrison ED, et al. Differences in hepatic phenotype between hemochromatosis patients with *HFE* C282Y homozygosity and other *HFE* genotypes. J Clin Gastroenterol 2009;43(6):569–73.
3. Adams PC, Reboussin DM, Barton JC, et al. Hemochromatosis and iron-overload screening in a racially diverse population. N Engl J Med 2005;352(17):1769–78.
4. European Association For The Study Of The Liver. EASL clinical practice guidelines for HFE hemochromatosis. J Hepatol 2010;53(1):3–22.
5. Allen KJ, Gurrin LC, Constantine CC, et al. Iron-overload-related disease in *HFE* hereditary hemochromatosis. N Engl J Med 2008;358(3):221–30.
6. Gleeson F, Ryan E, Barrett S, et al. Clinical expression of haemochromatosis in Irish C282Y homozygotes identified through family screening. Eur J Gastroenterol Hepatol 2004;16(9):859–63.
7. Bulaj ZJ, Ajioka RS, Phillips JD, et al. Disease-related conditions in relatives of patients with hemochromatosis. N Engl J Med 2000;343(21):1529–35.
8. Poullis A, Moodie SJ, Ang L, et al. Routine transferrin saturation measurement in liver clinic patients increases detection of hereditary haemochromatosis. Ann Clin Biochem 2003;40(Pt 5):521–7.
9. Pietrangelo A. Genetics, genetic testing, and management of hemochromatosis: 15 years since hepcidin. Gastroenterology 2015;149(5):1240–51.
10. Bonkovsky HL, Poh-Fitzpatrick M, Pimstone N, et al. Porphyria cutanea tarda, hepatitis C, and HFE gene mutations in North America. Hepatology 1998;27(6): 1661–9.
11. Beutler E, Felitti VJ, Koziol JA, et al. Penetrance of 845G–>A (C282Y) HFE hereditary haemochromatosis mutation in the USA. Lancet 2002;359(9302):211–8.
12. Powell LW, Dixon JL, Ramm GA, et al. Screening for hemochromatosis in asymptomatic subjects with or without a family history. Arch Intern Med 2006;166(3): 294–301.
13. Gordeuk VR, Reboussin DM, McLaren CE, et al. Serum ferritin concentrations and body iron stores in a multicenter, multiethnic primary-care population. Am J Hematol 2008;83(8):618–26.
14. Morrison ED, Brandhagen DJ, Phatak PD, et al. Serum ferritin level predicts advanced hepatic fibrosis among U.S. patients with phenotypic hemochromatosis. Ann Intern Med 2003;138(8):627–33.
15. Deugnier Y, Turlin B. Pathology of hepatic iron overload. Semin Liver Dis 2011; 31(3):260–71.
16. Banerjee R, Pavlides M, Tunnicliffe EM, et al. Multiparametric magnetic resonance for the non-invasive diagnosis of liver disease. J Hepatol 2014;60(1): 69–77.

17. Nelson JE, Wilson L, Brunt EM, et al. Relationship between pattern of hepatic iron deposition and histologic severity in nonalcoholic fatty liver disease. Hepatology 2011;53(2):448–57.
18. Lv T, Li X, Zhang W, et al. Recent advance in the molecular genetics of Wilson disease and hereditary hemochromatosis. Eur J Med Genet 2016;59(10):532–9.
19. Milman N, Pederson P, a Steig T, et al. Clinically overt hereditary hemochromatosis in Denmark 1948-1985: epidemiology, factors of significance for long-term survival and causes of death in 179 patients. Ann Hematol 2001;80:737–44.
20. Fracanzani AL, Fargion S, Romano R, et al. Portal hypertension and iron depletion in patients with genetic hemochromatosis. Hepatology 1995;22(4):1127–31.
21. Bosma PJ, Chowdhury JR, Bakker C, et al. The genetic basis of the reduced expression of bilirubin UDP-glucuronosyltransferase I in Gilbert's syndrome. N Engl J Med 1995;333(18):1171–5.
22. Maruo Y, Nakahara S, Yanagi T. Genotype of *UGT1A1* and phenotype correlation between Crigler-Najjar syndrome type II and Gilbert syndrome. J Gastroenterol Hepatol 2016;31(2):403–8.
23. Bailey A, Robinson D, Dawson AM. Does Gilbert's exist? Lancet 1977;1(8018): 931–3.
24. Powell LW, Hemingway E, Billing BH, et al. Idiopathic unconjugated hyperbilirubinemia (Gilbert's syndrome). N Engl J Med 1967;277(21):1108–12.
25. Owens D, Evans J. Population studies on Gilbert's syndrome. J Med Genet 1975; 12(2):152–6.
26. Abboud RT, Nelson TN, Jung B, et al. Alpha$_1$-antitrypsin deficiency: clinical-genetic overview. Appl Clin Genet 2011;4:55–65.
27. Perlmutter DH, Brodsky JL, Balistreri WF, et al. Molecular pathogenesis of alpha-1-antitrypsin deficiency-associated liver disease: a meeting review. Hepatology 2007;45:1313–23.
28. Birrer P, McElvaney NG, Chang-Stroman LM, et al. α-1 antitrypsin deficiency and liver disease. J Inherit Metab Dis 1991;14(4):512–25.
29. Stoller JK, Aboussouan LS. A review of α1-antitrypsin deficiency. Am J Respir Crit Care Med 2012;185(3):246–59.
30. Esnault VLM, Testa A, Audrain M, et al. Alpha-1 antitrypsin genetic polymorphism in ANCA-positive systemic vasculitis. Kidney Int 1993;43(6):1329–32.
31. Smith KC, Su WPD, Pittelkow MR, et al. Clinical and pathologic correlations in 96 patients with panniculitis, including 15 patients with deficient levels of α$_1$-antitrypsin. J Am Acad Dermatol 1989;21:1192–6.
32. Hutchison DC. α1-antitrypsin deficiency in Europe: geographical distribution of Pi types S and Z. Respir Med 1998;92(3):367–77.
33. de Serres FJ, Blanco I. Prevalence of α1-antitrypsin deficiency alleles PI*S and PI*Z worldwide and effective screening for each of the five phenotypic classes PI*MS, PI*MZ, PI*SS, PI*SZ, and PI*ZZ: a comprehensive review. Ther Adv Respir Dis 2012;6(5):277–95.
34. Chu AS, Chopra KB, Perlmutter DH. Is severe progressive liver disease caused by alpha-1-antitrypsin deficiency more common in children or adults? Liver Transpl 2016;22(7):886–94.
35. Sveger T. Liver disease in alpha-1-antitrypsin deficiency detected by screening of 200,000 infants. N Engl J Med 1976;294(24):1316–21.
36. Eriksson S, Carlson J, Velez R. Risk of cirrhosis and primary liver cancer in alpha 1-antitrypsin deficiency. N Engl J Med 1986;314(12):736–9.
37. Lomas DA, Evans DL, Finch JT, et al. The mechanism of Z alpha 1-antitrypsin accumulation in the liver. Nature 1992;357(6379):605–7.

38. Hood JM, Koep LJ, Peters RL, et al. Liver transplantation for advanced liver disease with alpha-1-antitrypsin deficiency. N Engl J Med 1980;302(5):272–5.
39. Tanzi RE, Petrukhin K, Chernov I, et al. The Wilson disease gene is a copper transporting ATPase with homology to the Menkes disease gene. Nat Genet 1993;5(4):344–50.
40. Merle U, Schaefer M, Ferenci P, et al. Clinical presentation, diagnosis and long-term outcome of Wilson's disease: a cohort study. Gut 2007;56(1):115–20.
41. Roberts EA, Schilsky ML. Diagnosis and treatment of Wilson disease: an update. Hepatology 2008;47(6):2089–111.
42. Reilly M, Daly L, Hutchinson M. An epidemiological study of Wilson's disease in the Republic of Ireland. J Neurol Neurosurg Psychiatry 1993;56(3):298–300.
43. European Association for Study of Liver. EASL clinical practice guidelines: Wilson's disease. J Hepatol 2012;56(3):671–85.
44. Gow PJ, Smallwood RA, Angus PW, et al. Diagnosis of Wilson's disease: an experience over three decades. Gut 2000;446(3):415–9.
45. Sallie R, Katsiyiannakis L, Baldwin D, et al. Failure of simple biochemical indexes to reliably differentiate fulminant Wilson's disease from other causes of fulminant liver failure. Hepatology 1992;16(5):1206–11.
46. Schilsky ML, Scheinberg IH, Sternlieb I. Prognosis of Wilsonian chronic active hepatitis. Gastroenterology 1991;100(3):762–7.
47. Ferenci P, Caca K, Loudianos G, et al. Diagnosis and phenotypic classification of Wilson disease. Liver Int 2003;23(3):139–42.
48. Nicastro E, Ranucci G, Vajro P, et al. Re-evaluation of the diagnostic criteria for Wilson disease in children with mild liver disease. Hepatology 2010;52(6):1948–56.
49. Ferenci P, Steindl-Munda P, Vogel W, et al. Diagnostic value of quantitative hepatic copper determination in patients with Wilson's disease. Clin Gastroenterol Hepatol 2005;3(8):811–8.
50. Fleming CR, Dickson ER, Wahner HW, et al. Pigmented corneal rings in non-Wilsonian liver disease. Ann Intern Med 1977;86(3):285–8.
51. Scheinberg H, Gitlin D. Deficiency of ceruloplasmin in patients with hepatolenticular degeneration. Science 1952;116(3018):4484–5.
52. Stromeyer FW, Ishak KG. Histology of the liver in Wilson's disease. Am J Clin Pathol 1980;73(1):12–24.
53. Santos Silva EE, Sarles J, Buts JP, et al. Successful medical treatment of severely decompensated Wilson disease. J Pediatr 1996;128:285–7.
54. Jacquemin E. Progressive familial intrahepatic cholestasis. Clin Res Hepatol Gastroenterol 2012;36(Suppl 1):S26–35.
55. Strautnieks SS, Byrne JA, Pawlikowska L, et al. Severe bile salt export pump deficiency: 82 different ABCB11 mutations in 109 families. Gastroenterology 2008;134(4):1203–14.
56. Davit-Spraul A, Gonzales E, Baussan C, et al. Progressive familial intrahepatic cholestasis. Orphanet J Rare Dis 2009;4:1.
57. Hoerning A, Raub S, Dechene A, et al. Diversity of disorders causing neonatal cholestasis–the experience of a tertiary pediatric center in Germany. Front Pediatr 2014;2:65.
58. Fischler B, Papadogiannakis N, Nemeth A. Clinical aspects on neonatal cholestasis based on observations at a Swedish tertiary referral centre. Acta Paediatr 2001;90(2):171–8.

59. El-Guindi MA, Sira MM, Hussein MH, et al. Hepatic immunohistochemistry of bile transporters in progressive familial intrahepatic cholestasis. Ann Hepatol 2016; 15(2):222–9.
60. Jung C, Driancourt C, Baussan C, et al. Prenatal molecular diagnosis of inherited cholestatic disease. J Pediatr Gastroenterol Nutr 2007;44(4):453–8.
61. Davit-Spraul A, Fabre M, Branchereau S, et al. *ATP8B1* and *ABCB11* analysis in 62 children with normal gamma-glutamyl transferase progressive familial intrahepatic cholestasis (PFIC): phenotypic differences between PFIC1 and PFIC2 and natural history. Hepatology 2010;51(5):1645–55.
62. Harris MJ, Le Couteur DG, Arias IM. Progressive familial intrahepatic cholestasis: genetic disorders of biliary transporters. J Gastroenterol Hepatol 2005;20(6): 807–17.
63. Folvik G, Hilde O, Helge GO. Benign recurrent intrahepatic cholestasis: review and long-term follow-up of five cases. Scand J Gastroenterol 2012;47(4):482–8.
64. Tygstrup N, Steig BA, Juijn JA, et al. Recurrent familial intrahepatic cholestasis in the Faeroe Islands. Phenotypic heterogeneity but genetic homogeneity. Hepatology 1999;29(2):506–8.
65. Su K, Donaldson E, Sharma R. Novel treatment options for lysosomal acid lipase deficiency: critical appraisal of sebelipase alfa. Appl Clin Genet 2016;9:157–67.
66. Bernstein DL, Hulkova H, Bialer MG, et al. Cholesteryl ester storage disease: review of the findings in 135 reported patients with an underdiagnosed disease. J Hepatol 2013;58(6):1230–43.
67. Muntoni S, Wiebusch H, Jansen-Rust M, et al. Prevalence of cholesteryl ester storage disease. Arterioscler Thromb Vasc Biol 2007;27(8):1866–8.
68. Wolman M, Sterk VV, Gatt S, et al. Primary familial xanthomatosis with involvement and calcification of the adrenals. Report of two more cases in siblings of a previously described infant. Pediatrics 1961;28:742–57.
69. Scott SA, Liu B, Nazarenko I, et al. Frequency of the cholesteryl ester storage disease common *LIPA* E8SJM mutation (c.894G>A) in various racial and ethnic groups. Hepatology 2013;58(3):958–65.
70. Pisciotta L, Fresa R, Bellocchio A, et al. Cholesteryl ester storage disease (CESD) due to novel mutations in the *LIPA* gene. Mol Genet Metab 2009;97(2):143–8.
71. Hamilton J, Jones I, Srivastava R, et al. A new method for the measurement of lysosomal acid lipase in dried blood spots using the inhibitor Lalistat 2. Clin Chim Acta 2012;413(15–16):1207–10.
72. Civallero G, de Mari J, Bittar C, et al. Extended use of a selective inhibitor of acid lipase for the diagnosis of Wolman disease and cholesteryl ester storage disease. Gene 2014;539(1):154–6.

Genetics and Precision Medicine
Heritable Thoracic Aortic Disease

Erin Demo, MS, CGC[a], Christina Rigelsky, MS, CGC[b],
Andrea L. Rideout, MS, CCGC, CGC[c], Madeline Graf, MS, LCGC[d],
Mitchel Pariani, MS, LCGC[e], Ellen Regalado, MS, CGC[f],
Gretchen MacCarrick, MS, CGC[g,*]

KEYWORDS

- Aortic aneurysm • Aortic dissection • Marfan • Genetic counseling
- Heritable thoracic aortic disease (HTAD)

KEY POINTS

- Aortic aneurysm/dissection in a relatively young and healthy individual or in someone with a positive family history of similar disease or sudden unexplained death should prompt referral to cardiology and genetics specialties.
- Medical management of heritable thoracic aortic disease (HTAD) typically involves treatment with blood pressure-lowering medications (ie, β blockers or angiotensin receptor blockers) and activity modifications, including avoidance of isometric exercises and avoidance of exercising to the point of exhaustion.
- A genetic diagnosis guides timing of surgical intervention of aneurysm and imaging surveillance type, location, and frequency. It also helps providers address family member risk and nonvascular manifestations.
- There can be overlapping expression of aortic disease and other manifestations within and between HTADs, thus gene panel testing is an important part of the diagnostic process.

[a] Sibley Heart Center Cardiology, 2835 Brandywine Road, Suite 300, Atlanta, GA 30341, USA; [b] Genomic Medicine Institute, Cleveland Clinic, 9500 Euclid Avenue, NE50, Cleveland, OH 44195, USA; [c] IWK Health Centre, 5850 University Avenue, PO Box 9700, Halifax, Nova Scotia B3K 6R8, Canada; [d] Stanford Health Care, 900 Blake Wilbur Drive, 3rd floor, Stanford, CA 94305, USA; [e] Stanford School of Medicine, 300 Pasteur Drive, 2nd Floor, Room H2157, Stanford, CA 94305, USA; [f] Invitae, 1400 16th Street, San Francisco, CA 94103, USA; [g] Johns Hopkins School of Medicine, Blalock 1008, 600 North Wolfe Street, Baltimore, MD 21287, USA
* Corresponding author.
E-mail address: goswald1@jhmi.edu

Med Clin N Am 103 (2019) 1005–1019
https://doi.org/10.1016/j.mcna.2019.08.001
0025-7125/19/© 2019 Elsevier Inc. All rights reserved.

medical.theclinics.com

INTRODUCTION

Aortic disease is becoming more prevalent in the general population as advancements in diagnosis and surgical interventions have evolved. The incidence of thoracic aortic aneurysm and dissection is estimated at 16.3 per 100,000 per year for men and 9.1 per 100,000 per year in women.[1] Aortic dissection and rupture have a high morbidity and mortality; therefore the best prevention is identification of asymptomatic and at-risk individuals so that vascular screening and elective surgery can be performed. There are many different causes of thoracic aortic aneurysm and dissection, including genetic and nongenetic factors. This review focuses on the heritable nature of this disease.

When to Suspect a Genetic Cause

It is important to consider both genetic and nongenetic factors that may have contributed to a patient's aortic aneurysm or dissection.

Nongenetic risk factors for aortic aneurysms and dissection can include[2–4]:

- Concurrent cardiovascular risk factors: long-standing/uncontrolled hypertension, atherosclerosis, and dyslipidemia
- Life events and lifestyle: pregnancy, extreme weight lifting, smoking, and cocaine use
- Inflammatory or infectious disease: autoimmune such as giant cell arteritis, Takayasu arteritis, and Bechet disease, or bacterial causes infections such as syphilis and tuberculosis
- Advanced age

Certain features suggest heritable thoracic aortic disease (HTAD), which can either be isolated (aorta only; nonsyndromic) or syndromic (involving other body systems such as the ocular or musculoskeletal systems). Aortopathy is more likely to be genetic when the affected individual is younger than 50 to 60 years old and/or has a family history of a first- or second-degree relative with aortic aneurysm or dissection.[5] A family history of sudden unexplained death or certain accidental deaths (such as motor vehicle accidents or drowning) should heighten suspicion for HTAD.

Joint hypermobility, which is a common feature seen in 10% of the general population, can be associated with aortopathy. However, the genetic causes of isolated hypermobility are largely unknown.[6] Joint hypermobility can also be commonly seen with other comorbidities including chronic pain, orthostatic intolerance, and gastrointestinal dysmotility. Individuals with hypermobility should consider an echocardiogram and referral for genetics evaluation if aortic dilation is present.

Of note, individuals who present with isolated brain aneurysms, coronary artery dissections, and/or other arterial dissections, especially when young, should be referred for genetics evaluation, because some HTADs can show variable expression with minimal aortic disease, but presence of other artery aneurysms/dissections.

Clinical Evaluations for Heritable Thoracic Aortic Disease

The workup for HTAD should ideally occur in a multidisciplinary genetics or cardiology clinic specializing in aortopathies. When there is a family history of HTAD, it is important to remember that even within a family there can be wide variability of clinical features and age of onset. In general, all first-degree family members of anyone with aortic aneurysm/dissection should have echocardiogram screening (unless the aneurysm has a clearly defined nongenetic cause).

Cardiology assessment should include echocardiogram with specific assessment of aortic valve annulus, mid-sinuses of Valsalva, sinotubular junction and ascending aortic diameters, aortic valve morphology, mitral valve disease, and other measurements of heart size and function (**Fig. 1**). History of congenital heart disease such as patent ductus arteriosus (PDA), mitral valve prolapse, or atrioventricular septal defects should also be considered.

Based on physical examination and medical or family history, a baseline computed tomography angiogram (CTA) or magnetic resonance angiogram (MRA) from head to pelvis, may be considered for detection of aortic or arterial aneurysms and tortuosity (especially of the carotid or vertebral arteries). Tortuosity is suggestive of HTAD and also a prognostic factor for dissection.[7]

Ophthalmology evaluation should be performed to document syndromic features such as ectopia lentis (Marfan syndrome [MFS]), esotropia, glaucoma, retinal detachment, cataract, high myopia, and iris flocculi (suggestive of *ACTA2* mutations).

Genetic Evaluation for Heritable Thoracic Aortic Disease: Proband

Genetic evaluation can play a crucial role in determining a patient's risk for aortic disease or dissection and risk to family members, through examination of personal or familial syndromic features (**Fig. 2**). Often, families can have great variability in extracardiac manifestations, and it is difficult to distinguish between syndromic versus nonsyndromic HTAD, highlighting the importance of HTAD gene panel testing in diagnosis.

Genetic testing continues to evolve as gene discovery rapidly develops. At present, over 30 genes have been associated with HTAD and more are expected to be identified.[8] Genetic testing panels are often the most useful and economical

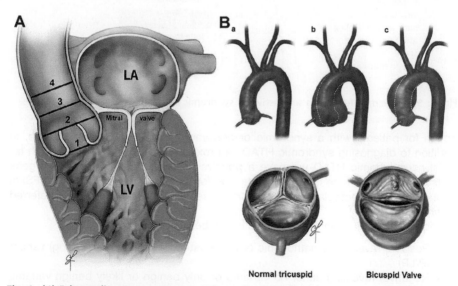

Fig. 1. (*A*) Echocardiogram assessment. Echocardiogram should assess the following diameters: 1, aortic valve annulus; 2, mid-sinuses of Valsalva; 3, sinotubular junction; and 4, ascending aorta. This will allow for an aortic profile to determine morphology of aorta. (*B*) a, normal aorta; b, aortic root aneurysm; c, ascending aortic aneurysm. The images show aortic valve morphology (tricuspid vs bicuspid). (Reprinted with permission, Cleveland Clinic Center for Medical Art & Photography © 2019. All Rights Reserved.)

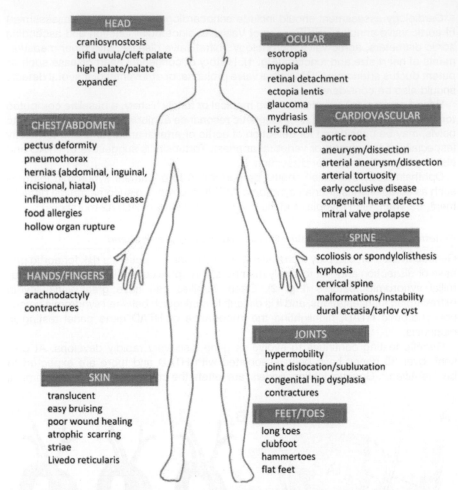

HEAD
craniosynostosis
bifid uvula/cleft palate
high palate/palate
expander

OCULAR
esotropia
myopia
retinal detachment
ectopia lentis
glaucoma
mydriasis
iris flocculi

CARDIOVASCULAR
aortic root
aneurysm/dissection
arterial aneurysm/dissection
arterial tortuosity
early occlusive disease
congenital heart defects
mitral valve prolapse

CHEST/ABDOMEN
pectus deformity
pneumothorax
hernias (abdominal, inguinal,
incisional, hiatal)
inflammatory bowel disease
food allergies
hollow organ rupture

SPINE
scoliosis or spondylolisthesis
kyphosis
cervical spine
malformations/instability
dural ectasia/tarlov cyst

HANDS/FINGERS
arachnodactyly
contractures

JOINTS
hypermobility
joint dislocation/subluxation
congenital hip dysplasia
contractures

SKIN
translucent
easy bruising
poor wound healing
atrophic scarring
striae
Livedo reticularis

FEET/TOES
long toes
clubfoot
hammertoes
flat feet

Fig. 2. Systemic manifestations suggestive of syndromic heritable thoracic aortic disease.

option for patients with a syndromic or nonsyndromic thoracic aortic disease. In addition to diagnosing syndromic HTAD, approximately 30% of individuals with familial nonsyndromic HTAD will have a positive result on current aortopathy gene testing panels.[8] With the exception of testing for the single gene *FBN1* (for MFS) in an individual with ectopia lentis and aortic disease, panel testing is the preferred testing method.

Genetic testing is nuanced. Test results can be:

- Positive, revealing a pathogenic or likely pathogenic (disease-causing) variant (P/LP)
- Negative, revealing either no variants or only benign or likely benign variants (B/LB)
- Variant of unknown significance (VUS), in which not enough is yet known about the variant to classify it as either P/LP or B/LB

In addition, panel testing may include genes for disorders that do not have aneurysmal disease, but overlap with the skeletal features of aneurysm syndromes. An example of genes and disorders on a current aortopathy gene panel is shown in **Fig. 3** and demonstrates the complexity of testing. Interpretation of variants compared with patient's clinical features as well as coordination of familial evaluations either via genetic testing or through clinical evaluation can be burdensome, especially in the case of VUS. Thus, genetics professionals who can interpret testing results and help with familial communication and review of records can be very helpful in coordination of care.

Rarely, patients with severe thoracic aortic disease and negative panel testing may need whole-exome testing to help identify the genetic cause. This is typically reserved for patients who are severely affected at a very young age, have extra-aortic manifestations, or families with multiple affected members. This is best managed by a genetics professional.

Individuals who have negative genetic testing could still have a heritable cause for their HTAD, but fall into the large percentage of cases in whom we cannot yet identify the genetic cause.

Genetic Evaluation for Heritable Thoracic Aortic Disease: Family Members

Most known HTAD conditions are inherited in an autosomal dominant pattern, conferring a 50% risk of recurrence to offspring and possibly parents and siblings. Family members of individuals with HTAD should be offered genetic counseling and consider genetic testing once a P/LP variant is detected in an affected family member. In families in which no P/LP variant is identified, cardiology evaluation with echocardiogram should be performed, with consideration of CTA/MRA based on cardiology evaluation. If aortic measurements are within normal limits, repeat evaluation should be considered every 2 to 5 years.[9]

Management of Heritable Thoracic Aortic Disease

In the past 10 years recognition and more specialized recommendations for management of HTAD have progressed considerably. Randomized controlled studies for management in this population are still rare, but what exists has been extrapolated across HTAD. The underlying genetic cause plays an important role in the management of HTAD conditions.

Surveillance
Ongoing cardiovascular surveillance is essential for individuals with HTAD. Baseline and (minimally) yearly echocardiogram imaging is indicated. More frequent imaging may be necessary as the aorta increases in size or approaches surgical threshold. Additional imaging of the aorta and/or arterial tree with CTA or MRA may be necessary. Patients who have had aortic surgery still require ongoing screening including the portion of the aorta beyond the repair.

Medical management
Strict blood pressure control is essential for patients with HTAD. The goal is less than 130/80.[10] β Blockers have been the mainstay of treatment for individuals with HTAD.[10] However, recent years have revealed angiotensin receptor blockers as reasonable alternative therapy or as complementary therapy to β blockers.[11] Other considerations include optimization of lipid values and smoking cessation as necessary. Some medications may have a greater risk profile for patients with HTAD, including stimulant medication (some attention deficit hyperactivity disorder medications and decongestants), fluoroquinolones, and vasoconstrictors, and therefore need personalized decision making before prescribing.[12,13]

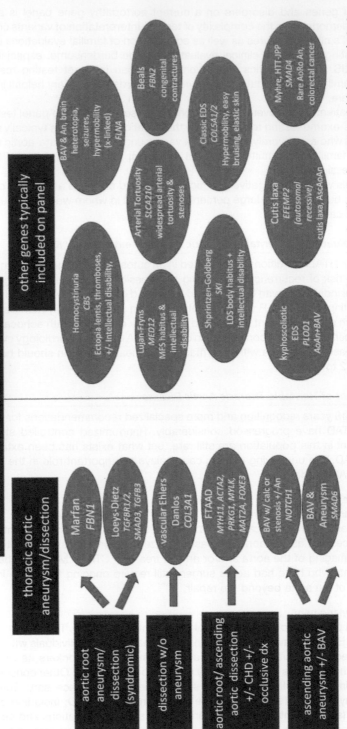

Fig. 3. Organization of genes and disorders tested for an example aortopathy gene panel (gene panels will vary by commercial laboratory). AoAn, aortic aneurysm; AscAoAn, ascending aortic aneurysm; BAV, bicuspid aortic valve; calc, calcification; CHD, congenital heart disease; EDS, Ehlers-Danlos syndrome; FTAAD, familial thoracic aortic aneurysm disease; LDS, Loeys-Dietz syndrome; MFS, Marfan syndrome.

Exercise recommendations
Exercise recommendations for HTAD are dependent on multiple factors including genetics, physical characteristics, and presence of aortic disease. Maintaining an active lifestyle is beneficial for overall health and mental well-being. In general, individuals with HTAD are advised to avoid activities that have high dynamic force, high static force (such as boxing, ice hockey, or wrestling) and that put them at higher chance of collision.[14] Isometric exercises (sit-ups, pushups, or weight lifting) are often contraindicated.

Management during pregnancy
Pre-pregnancy planning should be discussed with all women with HTAD of reproductive age. Imaging before pregnancy should include echocardiogram and updated MRA/CTA imaging if not performed recently. Women with HTAD are generally advised to consider repair of the aorta at 4.0 to 4.5 cm if they would like to get pregnant, because the risk associated with aortic dissection increases above 4.0 cm.[9]

Pregnancy and the postpartum period is a time for close surveillance in individuals with HTAD. Minimally, an echocardiogram should be performed during each trimester. Close evaluation in the postpartum period is equally as important because of the higher risk associated with dissection in this time period.[15,16] Women with HTAD should be followed by an obstetrician experienced in high risk situations, and a plan should be made for delivery at a center that has cardiothoracic or vascular surgery available. Consultation with an anesthesiologist should be made in advance of delivery so that a plan is in place to control pain while keeping blood pressure as low as possible. In syndromic HTAD, pre-pregnancy imaging should be used to assess for dural ectasia, which is important for anesthesiology considerations. Elective C-section is the most common mode of delivery for women with HTAD but can be personalized based on individual circumstances; assisted vaginal delivery may be considered. It is important for women to be counseled about the symptoms of dissection and advised to seek medical attention even if they have previously had an aortic repair, because risk associated with dissection in the descending aorta exists.[15]

In families where the pathogenic variant for HTAD is known in the affected parent, the family should be counseled on autosomal dominant inheritance and 50% chance of offspring being affected. Preimplantation genetic diagnosis, chorionic villus sampling, or amniocentesis to test the pregnancy is available. In addition, many families may choose to test the infant in the postnatal period.

Surgical decision making
The underlying genetic cause for HTAD is a guiding principle in timing of surgical intervention, but is still only one piece of information that must be considered. The surgical threshold based on gene is a guide, but should be personalized based on findings in the individual patient or family. Factors that could indicate need for early invention include: increased rate of progression (>0.5 cm/y increase in diameter), increasing aortic regurgitation, family history of dissection at small diameters, in patients with Loeys-Dietz syndrome (LDS), arterial tortuosity, and in women with small body surface area.[17] Conversely, waiting longer may be considered when there is favorable family history, including family members who have been able to be repaired without dissection at larger sizes or there has been stable dilatation for many years.

Valve-sparing aortic root replacement procedures are favored over mechanical graft, particularly in the young, to avoid the need for anticoagulation with an artificial valve.[9] Often, the choice of valve-sparing versus replacement is made by the surgeon physically examining the valve on intervention.

Open procedures are preferred over endovascular repairs, particularly for patients with heritable connective tissue diseases.[18] Endovascular stents may be considered as a bridge to an open repair in an emergency situation or in combination with Dacron grafts, in which the stent graft has a landing zone within the Dacron graft. Prophylactic aortic surgery should be performed in centers with high volume and with surgeons experienced in multiple techniques to ensure the most personalized plan for each patient.[9]

Examples of Heritable Thoracic Aortic Disease

There are many different genetic causes of HTAD, each having their own unique clinical manifestations (**Table 1**).

Marfan syndrome

MFS is caused by pathogenic variants in the *FBN1* gene that cause defects in the fibrillin-1 protein, a major component of the extracellular membrane, giving structural integrity and elastic properties to connective tissue.

Cardiovascular features of MFS include aortic root aneurysm or dissection and mitral valve prolapse. Rarely is there aneurysmal disease outside of the aorta. The revised Ghent criteria (2010) placed increased emphasis on genetic testing results and family history, along with criteria in the ocular (ectopia lentis), cardiovascular, and skeletal systems[19](**Fig. 4**). In MFS, prophylactic aortic root replacement is recommended when the aortic root reaches 5 cm, or when there is rapid growth of greater than 5 mm per year, but other indications such as family history, valve function, and severity of noncardiac features may affect surgical decision making. Mitral valve prolapse may also progress in severity requiring surgical intervention.

Routine ophthalmology evaluations are indicated with referrals to other specialists as needed (orthopedics, pain management, neurology [headaches or dural ectasia], endocrinology [low bone density]). Yearly echocardiograms should be performed with MRA or CTA of the entire aorta (chest, abdomen, and pelvis) performed every few years in adulthood or yearly if there is chronic dissection.

Loeys-Dietz syndrome

LDS was first attributed to pathogenic variants in the transforming growth factor beta (TGF-β) receptor 1 and 2 genes (*TGFBR1* and *TGFBR2*).[20] Subsequently, 3 additional genes in the TGF-β pathway have been described as causative of LDS (*TGFB2*, *TGFB3*, and *SMAD3*).[12] Observational studies reveal that some of these genetic defects lead to aortic dissection at aortic root diameters less than 5.0, and in some cases prophylactic aortic root surgery is recommended at diameters as small as 4.0 cm.[12]

Individuals with LDS may present with similar musculoskeletal features as MFS, but with a few distinct differences: arterial tortuosity, hypertelorism, broad/bifid uvula or cleft palate, craniosynostosis, clubfoot, and other cardiac defects (bicuspid aortic valve [BAV], ventricular septal defect, and PDA). Importantly, patients with LDS can have aneurysms and dissections throughout the arterial tree, necessitating routine head to pelvis MRA/CTA imaging. Cervical spine stability needs to be evaluated through flexion-extension radiographs of the neck. There is also increased prevalence of allergic (food and seasonal) disease and inflammatory gastrointestinal disease (eosinophilic disease and, rarely, inflammatory bowel disease) in LDS.[12] Referrals to orthopedics, pain management, neurology, gastroenterology, pulmonary, and ophthalmology should be performed as indicated.

Bicuspid aortic valve and aneurysm

BAV is the most common congenital heart defect, with an incidence of 2% of the population.[21] Some patients with nonsyndromic BAV develop aortic aneurysms most

Table 1
Comparison of selected heritable thoracic aortic disease disorders

	Marfan Syndrome	Loeys-Dietz Syndrome	Vascular Ehlers-Danlos Syndrome	FTAAD: Familial Thoracic Aortic Aneurysm Disease
Vascular				
Aortic root aneurysm	+	++	−	+; reduced penetrance
Aortic dissection	+	++	++	++
Arterial dissection	Rare	++	++	−
Arterial tortuosity	Rare	Common	Rare	Rare
Congenital heart defects	Rare	+	Rare	BAV, PDA
Skeletal				
Arachnodactyly	++	+	−	−
Dolichostenomelia	++	+	−	−
Pectus deformities	++	+	−	−
Scoliosis	++	+	Rare	−
Joint laxity	−	++	Small joint	−
Clubfoot	−	+	+	−
Cervical spine malformations	−	+	−	−
Facial				
Craniosynostosis	−	+	−	−
Hypertelorism	−	+	−	−
Cleft palate/bifid uvula	−	+	−	−
Skin				
Easy bruising	−	+	++	−
Atrophic scarring	−	+	++	−
Translucent skin	−	+	++	−
Eyes				
Ectopia lentis	+	−	−	−
Esotropia/strabismus	+	++	−	−
Retinal detachment	+	Rare	−	−
Mydriasis	−	−	−	+
Other				
Pneumothorax	+	Rare	++	−
Hollow organ rupture	−	Rare	++	−
Allergic/GI inflammatory disease	−	++	−	−
Strokes or occlusive disease	−	−	−	+

Abbreviations: BAV, bicuspid aortic valve; GI, gastrointestinal; PDA, patent ductus arteriosus.

commonly in the ascending aorta, but aneurysmal disease can occur in the root and transverse arch, with a tubular appearance.[22] Because of variable expressivity, family members may also present with BAV, BAV and aneurysm, aneurysm alone, or more rarely, severe left-sided heart defects such as hypoplastic left heart or coarctation

Without family history (FH)
(1) Ao (Z≥2) AND EL = MFS
(2) Ao (Z≥2) AND FBN1 = MFS
(3) Ao (Z≥2) AND Syst (≥7pts) = MFS
(4) EL AND FBN1 with known Ao=MFS

In presence of family history (FH) First degree family member affected
(5) EL AND FH of MFS = MFS
(6) Syst (≥7 pts) AND FH of MFS= MFS
(7) Ao (Z≥2 above 20 yrs old, ≥3 below 20 yrs) + FH
of MFS = MFS

Systemic score

Feature	Value
Wrist AND thumb sign	3
Wrist OR thumb sign	1
Pectus Carinatum deformity	2
Pectus excavatum or chest asymmetry	1
Hindfoot deformity	2
Plain flat foot (pes planus)	1
Pneumothorax	2
Dural Ectasia	2
Protrusio Acetabulae	2
Reduced upper segment/lower segment AND increased Arm span/Height ratios	1
Scoliosis or thoracolumbar kyphosis	1
Reduced elbow extension	1
3/5 facial features	1
Skin striae	1
Myopia	1
Mitral valve prolapse	1
(positive =7 or greater)	TOTAL

Fig. 4. Criteria for Marfan syndrome (revised Ghent criteria 2010). Ao, aortic diameter at the sinuses of Valsalva above indicated Z score or aortic root dissection; EL, ectopia lentis; FBN1, fibrillin mutation; FH, family history; MFS, Marfan syndrome; Syst, systemic score; Z, Z score.

of the aorta. The heritable nature of BAV has been validated in studies indicating genetic factors with reduced penetrance are at play.[23] Only 2 Mendelian genes have been discovered to date, NOTCH1 and SMAD6.[24] NOTCH1 has also been associated with early onset valve calcification and both left-sided and right-sided heart defects.[25] Most patients with BAV do not have the syndromic findings of MFS or LDS, however, can present with mild connective tissue disorder features, thus individuals with BAV and aneurysm do benefit from genetics evaluation to discuss the pros and cons of genetic testing and familial screening.

Regular echocardiogram imaging of the ascending aorta and the valve structure and function are indicated in any patient diagnosed with BAV, and surgery to replace the aorta is typically recommended at aortic dimensions around 5.0 to 5.5 cm.[8]

Vascular Ehler-Danlos syndrome

Vascular Ehlers-Danlos syndrome (vEDS) is caused by pathogenic variants in the COL3A1 gene and is characterized by vascular, cutaneous, and hollow organ tissue fragility. Individuals with vEDS have thin, translucent skin that bruises easily. There may be aortic or arterial dissection without preceding aneurysm. Hollow organ rupture (commonly bowel rupture) can occur. Many individuals with vEDS also have a characteristic facial appearance: pinched nose, thin upper lip, small chin, and prominent eyes. They can have spontaneous pneumothorax, hypermobility of the finger joints, and gingival bleeding and recession. vEDS may first become apparent in childhood with easy bruising, easily visible veins skin, clubfoot, and congenital dislocation of the hips; however, without a family history, the identification is often made much later with an event such as aortic rupture, pneumothorax, or spontaneous bowel rupture.[26]

Table 2
Rare causes of heritable thoracic aortic disease

Disorder/Gene	Inheritance	Distinctive Features	Cardiovascular Manifestations
Filamin A (*FLNA*)	X-linked	• Periventricular nodular heterotopias (PVNH) on MRI • Epilepsy • Male lethality	• HTAD • PDA, PFO, VSD • BAV/dysplastic valve • Mitral valve disease
Biglycan (*BGN*)	X-linked	• Hypertelorism • Short stature • Short, spatulate fingers	• HTAD
Shprintzen-Goldberg (*SKI*)	Autosomal dominant (de novo)	• Intellectual disability • Craniosynostosis • Clubfoot • Marfanoid habitus • C1-C2 vertebral abnormality	• HTAD (mild) • MVP • Neck artery tortuosity (rare)
Arterial tortuosity syndrome (*SLC2A10*)	Autosomal recessive	• Elongated face with beaked nose • Soft, doughy skin • Hernias: diaphragmatic, inguinal, abdominal • Muscle hypoplasia • Corneal thinning	• HTAD (mild; rare) • Focal stenosis of pulmonary arteries and aorta • Widespread arterial tortuosity • Risk for ischemic cerebrovascular events
Cutis laxa type 1B (*EFEMP2*)	Autosomal recessive	• Cutis laxa (variable) • Hypertelorism • Dysplastic ears • Diaphragmatic or inguinal hernias • Muscle hypoplasia	• HTAD (severe) • Focal stenosis of pulmonary arteries and aorta • Widespread arterial tortuosity • Risk for ischemic cerebrovascular events
SMAD4 disease • Juvenile polyposis/ heritable hemorrhagic telangiectasia (JPP-HHT) • Myhre syndrome	Autosomal dominant	JPP-HHT: • Arteriovenous malformations (cerebral, lung) • Epistaxis • Telangiectasias • GI hamartomatous polyps (risk for cancer) Myhre: • Short stature with skeletal anomalies on radiography • Intellectual disability/ autism • Laryngotracheal stenosis • Dysmorphic features	JPP-HHT: • HDAT (rare) Myhre: • Atrioventricular septal defects • Aortic/mitral valve stenosis • Left-sided obstruction defects • Pericardial effusion and fibrosis • Restrictive cardiomyopathy

Abbreviations: BAV, bicuspid aortic valve; GI, gastrointestinal; HTAD, heritable thoracic aneurysm disease; MVP, mitral valve prolapse; PDA, patent ductus arteriosus; PFO, patent foramen ovale; VSD, ventricular septal defect.

Many suggest that surveillance with detailed assessment of the arterial tree (head to pelvis MRA or CTA) should be performed yearly or every few years, although there is not consensus on this.[26] Tissue fragility leading to a tendency toward hemorrhage and poor wound healing can complicate surgeries, thus invasive or cosmetic procedures should be pursued with caution and performed by a surgeon experienced with connective tissue disorders. It is recommended to also have strict bowel control through diet or gentle laxative to reduce risk of bowel rupture.

Turner syndrome

Turner syndrome is a chromosome disorder in women caused by partial or complete loss of one of the X chromosomes. The incidence of Turner syndrome is approximately 1 in 2000 births. Women with Turner syndrome present with short stature, learning difficulties, delayed puberty, and infertility. Cardiac disease occurs in 30% to 45% of women with Turner syndrome, including BAV, aortic coarctation, aortic stenosis, and aortic aneurysm. Ischemic heart disease and hypertension are also common.[27]

Aortic dissection occurs in 1% to 2% of individuals with Turner syndrome, with two-thirds of dissections occurring in the ascending aorta and one-third in the descending aorta. Dissections typically occur in a patient's fourth to sixth decade.[28] Risk factors for aortic dissection for women with Turner syndrome include: coarctation of the aorta, BAV, aortic valve dysfunction, pregnancy, and hypertension. When assessing a woman with Turner syndrome for aortic surgery, it is important to note that there are Turner syndrome-specific Z scores (PMID: 28328137).[29]

Familial Thoracic Aortic Aneurysms and Dissections

Individuals may present with young onset or familial thoracic aortic disease with no or minimal features of a syndromic HTAD, generally referred to as familial thoracic aortic aneurysm and dissection. Most of the genes in this category encode proteins involved in smooth muscle contraction: *ACTA2* (α-actin), *MYH11* (myosin heavy chain), *MYLK* (myosin light chain kinase), and *PRKG1* (cGMP-dependent protein kinase).[30] These genetic disorders mostly present with thoracic aneurysm and dissection (both Stanford type A and B) with specific additional features, such as cerebrovascular and/or coronary artery disease, iris flocculi, multisystemic smooth muscle dysfunction syndrome (*ACTA2*), patent ductus arteriosus (*ACTA2* and *MYH11*), and aortic dissection with minimal enlargement (*MYLK*). Age of onset and aortic disease presentation can be variable.

Rare Genetic Considerations in Heritable Thoracic Aortic Disease

Less-common genetic syndromes associated with aneurysm or cardiac disease are also on the aneurysm gene panel (**Table 2**). These disorders represent variable forms of inheritance, cardiovascular features, and other medical characteristics.[31–37]

SUMMARY

Genetic evaluation and diagnosis can have significant impact on an individual's health care including guidance for imaging surveillance, medical therapy, surgical intervention, and other, noncardiac, manifestations. Genetics professionals can help facilitate genetic testing and risk assessment for other family members. Early diagnosis and management can potentially prevent catastrophic outcomes of sudden death due to aortic and arterial dissection. Genetic counseling and testing should be included in routine workup in HTAD without clear vasculitis or lifestyle/environmental cause.

REFERENCES

1. Olsson C, Thelin S, Ståhle E, et al. Thoracic aortic aneurysm and dissection: increasing prevalence and improved outcomes reported in a nationwide population-based study of more than 14,000 cases from 1987 to 2002. Circulation 2006;114(24):2611–8.
2. Watts RA, Robson J. Introduction, epidemiology and classification of vasculitis. Best Pract Res Clin Rheumatol 2018;32(1):3–20.
3. Elsayed R, Cohen R, Fleischman F, et al. Acute type A aortic dissection. Cardiol Clin 2017;35:331–45.
4. Deipolyi AR, Czaplicki CD, Oklu R. Inflammatory and infectious aortic diseases. Cardiovasc Diagn Ther 2018;8(Suppl 1):S61–70.
5. Verhagen JMA, Kempers M, Cozijnsen L, et al. Expert consensus recommendations on the cardiogenetic care for patients with thoracic aortic disease and their first-degree relatives. Int J Cardiol 2018;258:243–8.
6. Singh H, McKay M, Baldwin J, et al. Beighton scores and cut-offs across the lifespan: cross-sectional study of an Australian population. Rheumatology (Oxford) 2017;56(11):1857–64.
7. Morris SA. Arterial tortuosity in genetic arteriopathies. Curr Opin Cardiol 2015; 30(6):587–93.
8. Brownstein AJ, Kostiuk V, Ziganshin BA, et al. Genes associated with thoracic aortic aneurysm and dissection: 2018 update and clinical implications. Aorta (Stamford) 2018;6(1):13–20.
9. Hiratzka LF, Bakris GL, Beckman JA, et al. 2010 ACCF/AHA/AATS/ACR/ASA/ SCA/SCAI/SIR/STS/SVM guidelines for the diagnosis and management of patients with Thoracic Aortic Disease: a report of the American College of Cardiology Foundation/American Heart Association Task Force on Practice Guidelines, American Association for Thoracic Surgery, American College of Radiology, American Stroke Association, Society of Cardiovascular Anesthesiologists, Society for Cardiovascular Angiography and Interventions, Society of Interventional Radiology, Society of Thoracic Surgeons, and Society for Vascular Medicine. Circulation 2010;121(13):e266–369.
10. Whelton PK, Carey RM, Aronow WS. 2017 ACC/AHA/AAPA/ABC/ACPM/AGS/ APhA/ASH/ASPC/NMA/PCNA guideline for the prevention, detection, evaluation, and management of high blood pressure in adults: a report of the American College of Cardiology/American Heart Association Task Force on Clinical Practice Guidelines. Hypertension 2017;71:e13–115.
11. Teixido-Tura G, Forteza A, Rodriguez-Palomares J, et al. Losartan versus atenolol for prevention of aortic dilation in patients with Marfan syndrome. J Am Coll Cardiol 2018;72(14):1613–8.
12. MacCarrick G, Black JH 3rd, Bowdin S, et al. Loeys-Dietz syndrome: a primer for diagnosis and management. Genet Med 2014;16(8):576–87.
13. Pasternak B, Inghammar M, Svanstrom H. Fluoroquinolone use and risk of aortic aneurysm and dissection: nationwide cohort study. BMJ 2018;360:k678.
14. Levine BD, Baggish AL, Kovacs RJ, et al. Eligibility and disqualification recommendations for competitive athletes with cardiovascular abnormalities: task force 1: classification of sports: dynamic, static, and impact: a scientific statement from the American Heart Association and American College of Cardiology. Circulation 2015;132(22):e262–6.
15. Frise CJ, Pitcher A, Mackillop L. Loeys-Dietz syndrome and pregnancy: the first ten years. Int J Cardiol 2017;226:21–5.

16. Regalado ES, Guo DC, Estrera AL, et al. Acute aortic dissections with pregnancy in women with ACTA2 mutations. Am J Med Genet A 2014;164A(1):106–12.
17. Jondeau G, Ropers J, Regalado E, et al. International registry of patients carrying TGFBR1 or TGFBR2 mutations: results of the MAC (Montalcino Aortic Consortium). Circ Cardiovasc Genet 2016;9(6):548–58.
18. Bockler D, Meisenbacher K, Peters AS, et al. Endovascular treatment of genetically linked aortic diseases. Gefasschirurgie 2017;22(Suppl 1):1–7.
19. Loeys BL, Dietz HC, Braverman AC, et al. The revised Ghent nosology for the Marfan syndrome. J Med Genet 2010;47(7):476–85.
20. Loeys BL, Chen J, Neptune ER, et al. A syndrome of altered cardiovascular, craniofacial, neurocognitive and skeletal development caused by mutations in TGFBR1 or TGFBR2. Nat Genet 2005;37(3):275–81.
21. Ward C. Clinical significance of the bicuspid aortic valve. Heart 2000;83:81–5.
22. Fazel SS, Mallidi HR, Lee RS, et al. The aortopathy of bicuspid aortic valve disease has distinctive patterns and usually involves the transverse aortic arch. J Thorac Cardiovasc Surg 2008;135(4):901–7, 907.e1-2.
23. Cripe L, Andelfinger G, Martin LJ, et al. Bicuspid aortic valve is heritable. J Am Coll Cardiol 2004;44:138–43.
24. Tan HL, Glen E, Töpf A, et al. Nonsynonymous variants in the SMAD6 gene predispose to congenital cardiovascular malformation. Hum Mutat 2012;33(4): 720–7.
25. Kerstjens-Frederikse WS, van de Laar IM, Vos YJ, et al. Cardiovascular malformations caused by NOTCH1 mutations do not keep left: data on 428 probands with left-sided CHD and their families. Genet Med 2016;18(9):914–23.
26. Byers PH, Belmont J, Black J, et al. Diagnosis, natural history, and management in vascular Ehlers-Danlos syndrome. Am J Med Genet C Semin Med Genet 2017; 175(1):40–7.
27. Davenport ML. Turner syndrome. In: Cassidy SB, Allanson JE, editors. Management of genetic syndromes. 3rd edition. Hoboken (New Jersey): Wiley-Blackwell; 2010. p. 847–70.
28. Mortensen KH, Andersen NL, Gravholt CH. Cardiovascular phenotype in Turner syndrome—integrating cardiology, genetics and endocrinology. Endocr Rev 2012;33(50):677–714.
29. Prakash S, GenTAC Registry Investigators, Milewicz D. Turner syndrome-specific and general population Z-scores are equivalent for most adults with Turner syndrome. Am J Med Genet A 2017 Apr;173(4):1094–6.
30. Milewicz DM, Regalado E. Heritable thoracic aortic disease overview. In: Adam MP, Ardinger HH, Pagon RA, et al, editors. GeneReviews® [Internet]. Seattle (WA): University of Washington, Seattle; 1993–2019. Available at: https://www. ncbi.nlm.nih.gov/books/NBK1120/.
31. Chen MH, Choudhury S, Hirata M, et al. Thoracic aortic aneurysm in patients with loss of function Filamin A mutations: clinical characterization, genetics and recommendations. Am J Med Genet A 2018;176(2):337–50.
32. Meester JA, Vandeweyer G, Pintelon I, et al. Loss-of-function mutations in the X-linked biglycan gene cause a severe syndromic form of thoracic aortic aneurysms and dissections. Genet Med 2017;19(4):386–95.
33. Loeys B, De Paepe A, Urban Z. EFEMP2-related cutis laxa. In: Adam MP, Ardinger HH, Pagon RA, et al, editors. GeneReviews® [Internet]. Seattle (WA): University of Washington, Seattle; 1993–2019. Available at: https://www.ncbi. nlm.nih.gov/books/NBK54467/.

34. Beyens A, Albuisson J, Boel A, et al. Arterial tortuosity syndrome: 40 new families and literature review. Genet Med 2018;20(10):1236–45.
35. Schepers D, Doyle AJ, Oswald G, et al. The SMAD-binding domain of SKI: a hotspot for de novo mutations causing Shprintzen-Goldberg syndrome. Eur J Hum Genet 2015;23(2):224–8.
36. Lin AE, Michot C, Cormier-Daire V, et al. Gain-of-function mutations in SMAD4 cause a distinctive repertoire of cardiovascular phenotypes in patients with Myhre syndrome. Am J Med Genet A 2016;170(10):2617–31.
37. Renard M, Francis C, Ghosh R, et al. Clinical validity of genes for heritable thoracic aortic aneurysm and dissection. J Am Coll Cardiol 2018;72(6):605–15.

Symptomatic Joint Hypermobility

The Hypermobile Type of Ehlers-Danlos Syndrome and the Hypermobility Spectrum Disorders

Brad T. Tinkle, MD, PhD[a,*], Howard P. Levy, MD, PhD[b]

KEYWORDS

- Ehlers-Danlos syndrome • Hypermobility spectrum disorder • Joint hypermobility • Hypermobility syndrome • Joint pain • Orthostasis

KEY POINTS

- Joint hypermobility and generalized joint hypermobility can be quickly screened for.
- Joint hypermobility may be asymptomatic but alter biomechanics, and can cause activity-related pain, promote pain in other bodily sites, or portend future concerns.
- Joint hypermobility may be part of a heritable disorder of connective tissue.
- Systemic manifestations associated with joint hypermobility may be overt and should alert the practitioner to other areas of concern.

INTRODUCTION

Joint hypermobility is defined as excessive motion of a joint in the normal plane and is sometimes referred to as loose joints or double jointed. In contrast, joint laxity is used more often to refer to a joint that is unstable but is also sometimes used synonymously as loose ligaments or hyperlaxity. A joint can be lax but not hypermobile and vice

---

Disclosures: B.T. Tinkle is a paid consultant with Resolys Inc.; volunteer medical advisor to the Ehlers-Danlos Syndrome Society, Hypermobility Syndromes Association, and Ehlers-Danlos Syndrome UK; speaker's bureau of Alexion Pharmaceuticals; author of *Joint Hypermobility Handbook* and *Issues and Management of Joint Hypermobility Handbook*. H.P. Levy is a paid member of the medical advisory board of eviCore.

[a] Division of Medical Genetics, Peyton Manning Children's Hospital, 8402 Harcourt Road, Suite 300, Indianapolis, IN 46260, USA; [b] Division of General Internal Medicine, McKusick-Nathans Institute of Genetic Medicine, Johns Hopkins University, 10753 Falls Road, Suite 325, Baltimore, MD 21093, USA
* Corresponding author.
E-mail address: brad.tinkle@ascension.org

Med Clin N Am 103 (2019) 1021–1033
https://doi.org/10.1016/j.mcna.2019.08.002
0025-7125/19/Published by Elsevier Inc.

versa. However, such imprecise terminology results in confusion and the two terms are commonly used interchangeably. Generalized joint hypermobility (GJH) is defined as hypermobility affecting multiple joints, ideally involving all 4 limbs plus the axial skeleton.[1]

Using various scoring systems and across multiple populations, GJH can have a large range of prevalence of 2% to 57% or even sometimes higher.[2] Various scoring systems have been applied that use different sets of joints, measurements, and cut-offs. A recent comprehensive review found the Beighton scoring system (**Fig. 1**) the most reproducible but still with many shortcomings.[3] Advantages of the Beighton system include measuring a limited number of joints (9), being a quick in-office examination (<2 minutes), and good inter-rater reliability.[4,5]

Several confounding variables make the universal application of 1 scoring system problematic. Joint mobility varies with age, gender, training, injury, and racial/ethnic background.[6,7] This variability leads to controversy regarding the threshold for joint hypermobility. The original Beighton article used a threshold of 5 out of 9,[4] but scores of 4 or 6 (and sometimes lower) have been used or proposed in various settings.[7–9] Additional research is ongoing regarding age-specific and other demographic adjustments of the threshold for a positive Beighton score, as well as for development of more objective (but easy to perform) measures of GJH.

One key observation in a general US population of children and adolescents is that Beighton scores are statistically similar in prepubertal boys and girls, but female scores increase whereas male scores decrease during puberty.[10] This finding implies that joint mobility in general is increased or decreased respectively (not just the Beighton score) and, because the difference occurred only with puberty, that there is an effect of pubertal hormones on joint hypermobility. This effect may account for the large disproportion of symptomatic women compared with men (known as a sex-influenced trait) as well as the age of presentation for symptoms.[11] Anecdotally, the age of presentation of daily joint pain or dysfunction in women is more often after the onset of menses.

However, many people with joint hypermobility, including GJH, are asymptomatic. There are many theories about why one hypermobile person has pain whereas another may not, but there has been little substantiation.[12] The biomechanical concern about joint hypermobility is that any joint in the hypermobile range may be stressed and susceptible to repetitive use injury.[13,14] Joint stability depends on ligaments, muscles (and their associated tendons), and the joint capsule.[15] Hypermobility may result from

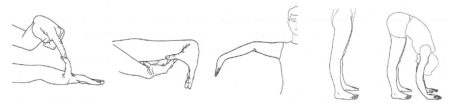

Fig. 1. The Beighton scoring system. The total possible score is 9, including 1 point for each of: hyperextension of either fifth finger metacarpophalangeal (MCP) joint beyond 90° (measured only at the MCP, not including the interphalangeal joints); apposition of either thumb to the ipsilateral forearm so that the thumb touches the skin; hyperextension of either elbow beyond 10°, as measured with a goniometer; hyperextension of either knee beyond 10°, as measured with a goniometer; forward flexion of the spine so that the palms lay flat on the floor directly in front of the feet, while knees are fully extended. (*Courtesy of* B. Juul-Kristensen, PhD, Odense, Denmark.)

deficiency of 1 or more of these structures. A hypermobile joint, regardless of the underlying cause, may depend more on musculotendinous function for stability, which may cause muscle strain, muscle spasm, tendonitis, and pain. The hypermobile joint can also alter the biomechanics of the body, causing compensatory changes and further strain. For example, the flexible flat foot can cause pronation and heel valgus, which can result in gait disturbance, knee pain, and back pain.[16–19]

CAUSES OF GENERALIZED JOINT HYPERMOBILITY

Like most human traits, joint hypermobility is a multifactorial condition resulting from a combination of environmental factors (eg, age, trauma, injury, conditioning, infection, inflammation) and multiple genetic factors, each contributing a small amount to the total phenotype. Joint hypermobility and GJH may also be part of many different heritable genetic syndromes. A search of Online Mendelian Inheritance in Man (OMIM; an extensive catalog of human genes and genetic disorders) for the term "joint hypermobility" returns more than 100 results; adding the term "joint laxity" returns almost 300 results.[20] Many of these are heritable disorders of connective tissue, such as Loeys-Dietz, Marfan, Stickler, and the Ehlers-Danlos syndromes (EDSs), or bone dysplasias, such as nail-patella syndrome, osteogenesis imperfecta, and achondroplasia. Neuromuscular disorders (leading to low muscle tone) and a variety of other genetic conditions (eg, Noonan syndrome, fragile X syndrome) also frequently manifest altered joint dynamics and joint hypermobility. Aside from EDS, most of these disorders present with other findings that can help with diagnosis, as long as the clinician remains alert for such findings. However, in EDS, joint hypermobility is often the most prominent feature. In addition, many patients with significant joint hypermobility (whether symptomatic or not) do not meet strict diagnostic criteria for any of the types of EDS or any other named condition but still are clearly outside the normal range of joint mobility and many have significant comorbidities. These patients should be classified as having hypermobility spectrum disorder (HSD) so as to validate their clinical status and help them receive necessary services[1]; they should not be labeled with EDS if they do not meet diagnostic criteria.[8] For the purpose of this article, the syndromes outside of EDS and HSD are not addressed, but the treatment of joint hypermobility itself varies little across conditions.

EHLERS-DANLOS SYNDROMES

EDS represents a group of 13 different but related heritable connective tissue disorders that have predominantly in common joint and skin manifestations (**Table 1**). The International Consortium on Ehlers-Danlos Syndromes updated the nosology and diagnostic criteria for all types of EDS in 2017.[8,21] Joint hypermobility, and in particularly GJH, is common to all types and the Beighton scoring system is recommended to assess this in all types. The skin texture varies from doughy to normal. The skin may also be stretchy and/or fragile (tearing easily), there may be delayed wound healing, and scars may be atrophic. The vascular type of EDS (vEDS) may also have a more translucent skin appearance. Many patients with joint hypermobility have other signs and symptoms, which help to differentiate between various connective tissue disorders such as Marfan, Stickler, or most of the types of EDS. However, the common presentation of predominant joint hypermobility and its complications but without overt clinical findings of a more specific diagnosis is likely to be in the category of the hypermobile type of EDS (hEDS) or HSD.

Confirmatory genetic testing is available for 12 of the 13 types of EDS. The underlying genetic causes for hEDS and for HSD remain unknown, so these diagnoses are

Table 1
Classification of the Ehlers-Danlos syndromes

EDS Type	Inheritance Pattern	Genes	Joint Hypermobility	Skin	Other Clinical Characteristics
Classic EDS	Autosomal dominant	COL5A1, COL5A2 Rare: COL1A1	Generalized	Stretchy, doughy, fragile, atrophic scars	—
Classiclike EDS	Autosomal recessive	TNXB	Generalized	Stretchy; velvety; without atrophic scars	Foot deformities; muscle weakness/atrophy
Cardiac-valvular EDS	Autosomal recessive	COL1A2	Generalized or limited to distal joints	Stretchy; fragile; atrophic scars	Progressive cardiac valve abnormalities
vEDS	Autosomal dominant	COL3A1 Rare: COL1A1	Small joints	Translucent, fragile; atrophic scars	Arterial or intestinal rupture; uterine rupture; carotid-cavernous sinus fistula
hEDS	Autosomal dominant	Unknown	Generalized	Mildly soft; mildly stretchy; mildly atrophic scars	—
Arthrochalasia EDS	Autosomal dominant	COL1A1, COL1A2	Generalized (severe); congenital hip dysplasia	Stretchy; fragile; atrophic scars	Hypotonia
Dermatosparaxis EDS	Autosomal recessive	ADAMTS2	Generalized	Stretchy; doughy; extreme fragility; atrophic scars	Characteristic facial features; growth retardation; short limbs, bladder or diaphragm rupture
Kyphoscoliotic EDS	Autosomal recessive	PLOD1, FKBP14	Generalized	Stretchy; fragile	Hypotonia; arterial rupture; early-onset kyphoscoliosis

Brittle-Cornea syndrome	Autosomal recessive	ZNF469, PRDM5	Distal joints, hip dysplasia	Soft; velvety; translucent	Thin cornea; blue sclerae; hearing loss
Spondylodysplastic EDS	Autosomal recessive	B4GALT7, B3GALT6, SLC39A13	Generalized or limited to distal joints	Stretchy; doughy; translucent	Short stature, hypotonia; bowing of long bones; developmental delay
Musculocontractural EDS	Autosomal recessive	CHST14, DSE	Multiple contractures; recurrent dislocations	Stretchy; fragile; atrophic scars; palmar wrinkling	Characteristic facial features; large hematomas
Myopathic EDS	Autosomal dominant or recessive	COL12A1	Distal joint hypermobility; proximal contractures	Doughy; atrophic scars	Hypotonia; developmental delay
Periodontal EDS	Autosomal dominant	C1R, C1S	Distal joints	Stretchy; fragile; atrophic scars	Severe periodontal disease; frequent infections

Adapted from Malfait F, Francomano C, Byers P, et al. The 2017 international classification of the Ehlers-Danlos syndromes. Am J Med Genet C Semin Med Genet 2017;175(1):10; with permission.

established on a clinical basis only. Rigorous application of the revised 2017 diagnostic criteria for hEDS (discussed later) and classification of those not meeting these criteria (nor criteria for any other condition) with HSD is expected to facilitate identification of the underlying genetic causes of hEDS.[8]

HYPERMOBILE EHLERS-DANLOS SYNDROME

Historically, people with GJH were often diagnosed with a spectrum of conditions such as familial joint laxity or benign joint hypermobility syndrome (BJHS). Familial joint laxity largely explained a heritable condition with joint hypermobility with or without other musculoskeletal issues, and is more descriptive than defining. BJHS was defined in 1967 by Kirk and colleagues[22] as a chronic condition with acute and often chronic pain, as well as recurring soft tissue injuries. BJHS was described in an adult population who have or had GJH. The older Villefranche diagnostic criteria for EDS originally described hEDS in a pediatric population of those having GJH with or without skin findings and other consequences, such as dislocations or pain.[23] Familial studies of those with symptomatic GJH made it apparent that the previously described hEDS under the Villefranche criteria presented itself as BJHS in an older adult population and the two descriptions were considered to represent a clinical continuum.[6,24,25] However, hEDS as a clinical diagnosis lacked specificity and a large undertaking to redefine hEDS clinically and genetically to enhance diagnostic specificity, pathophysiologic understanding, and management of this common condition continues to take place through the International Consortium on the Ehlers-Danlos Syndromes.[26] Therefore, hEDS was more recently redefined through a complicated set of more rigorous diagnostic criteria (**Box 1**). However, this makes the diagnosis in a primary care setting more challenging and further refinements of the criteria are likely in the near future.

MULTISYSTEMIC COMORBIDITIES AND MANAGEMENT

Many of those who are considered to have GJH may present with various manifestations. The most common, especially in patients with hEDS and HSD but often seen in hypermobile patients with other diagnoses, include joint subluxations/dislocations, periarticular pain, chronic diffuse pain, headaches, fatigue, postural dizziness, and/or gastrointestinal manifestations.[1,26]

JOINT HYPERMOBILITY AND INSTABILITY

Asymptomatic joint hypermobility may still need to be addressed, because this could be a precursor to future musculoskeletal issues. Many young children have asymptomatic joint hypermobility, manifesting as various postures such as W sitting and simple contortions. This constant stress on the joints may perpetuate joint laxity and cause muscle tension and future activity-related pain with repetitive tasks and/or exposure to heavy loads. This pain is often misinterpreted as so-called growing pains. Many adults with symptomatic joint hypermobility remember themselves as largely asymptomatic double-jointed children. Also remember that a hypermobile joint can sometimes alter the mechanics of other joints leading to pain, such as the aforementioned flexible flat foot leading to knee, hip, or lower back pain. Regardless of age, asymptomatic hypermobile persons would benefit from regular physical activity, instruction of proper ergonomics, and avoidance of extreme contorting.

Symptomatic joint hypermobility, instability, and periarticular pain should be addressed whether syndromic or nonsyndromic and regardless of how many or

---

Box 1
The diagnostic criteria for the hypermobile type of Ehlers-Danlos syndrome

The clinical diagnosis of hEDS needs the simultaneous presence of criteria 1 and 2 and 3.
Criterion 1: GJH with positive Beighton score[a]
- ≥6 for prepubertal children
- ≥5 for pubertal persons up to the age of 50 years
- ≥4 for those more than 50 years

Criterion 2: 2 or more among the following features (A, B, and C) must be present
    Feature A: 5 or more of the following systemic manifestations of a generalized connective tissue disorder
    1. Unusually soft or velvety skin
    2. Mild skin hyperextensibility, tested on the volar aspect of the forearm (not over extensor surfaces)
    3. Unexplained stretch marks (unrelated to puberty or weight change)
    4. Bilateral piezogenic papules of the heel
    5. Recurrent or multiple abdominal hernias (eg, umbilical, inguinal, crural)
    6. Atrophic scarring involving at least 2 sites
    7. Pelvic floor, rectal, and/or uterine prolapse in the absence of pregnancy or morbid obesity
    8. Dental crowding and high or narrow palate
    9. Arachnodactyly, defined by 1 or both of (i) positive wrist sign (Steinberg sign) on both sides; (ii) positive thumb sign (Walker sign) on both sides
    10. Arm span/height ratio ≥1.05
    11. Mitral valve prolapse, based on strict echocardiographic criteria
    12. Aortic root dilatation with Z-score greater than +2
    Feature B: positive family history, defined as 1 or more first-degree relatives independently meeting the current diagnostic criteria for hEDS.
    Feature C: at least 1 of the following musculoskeletal complications
    1. At least 3 months of daily pain in 2 or more limbs
    2. Chronic, widespread pain for at least 3 months
    3. Recurrent joint dislocations or frank joint instability, in the absence of trauma (a or b)
        a. Three or more atraumatic dislocations in the same joint or 2 or more atraumatic dislocations in 2 different joints occurring at different times
        b. Medical confirmation of atraumatic joint instability at 2 or more sites

Criterion 3: all the following prerequisites must be met
1. Absence of unusual skin fragility, which should prompt consideration of other types of EDS.
2. Exclusion of other heritable and acquired connective tissue disorders, including autoimmune rheumatologic conditions.
3. Exclusion of alternative diagnoses that may also include joint hypermobility by means of hypotonia and/or connective tissue laxity. Alternative diagnoses and diagnostic categories include, but are not limited to, neuromuscular disorders (eg, Bethlem myopathy), other hereditary disorders of connective tissue (eg, other types of EDS, Loeys-Dietz syndrome, Marfan syndrome), and skeletal dysplasias (eg, osteogenesis imperfecta). Exclusion of these considerations may be based on history, physical examination, and/or molecular genetic testing, as indicated.

[a] Note that a point may be added to the Beighton score if the 5-point questionnaire is positive (**Box 2**).

Adapted from Malfait F, Francomano C, Byers P, et al. The 2017 international classification of the Ehlers-Danlos syndromes. Am J Med Genet C Semin Med Genet 2017;175(1):8-26; with permission.

---

few joints are affected. Physical and occupational therapy is the mainstay of management. Although high-quality evidence is still lacking, the general approach typically includes techniques to reduce spasm (eg, relaxation, massage, hydrotherapy, stretching) and low-resistance/low-impact exercise designed to increase tone,

Box 2
The 5-point questionnaire

1. Can you now (or could you ever) place your hands flat on the floor without bending your knees?
2. Can you now (or could you ever) bend your thumb to touch your forearm?
3. As a child, did you amuse your friends by contorting your body into strange shapes or could you do the splits?
4. As a child or teenager, did your shoulder or kneecap dislocate on more than 1 occasion?
5. Do you consider yourself double jointed?

A yes answer to 2 or more questions suggests joint hypermobility with 80% to 85% sensitivity and 80% to 90% specificity.

Adapted from Hakim AJ, Grahame R. A simple questionnaire to detect hypermobility: an adjunct to the assessment of patients with diffuse musculoskeletal pain. Int J Clin Pract 2003;57(3):164; with permission.

stability, and endurance.[26,27] Hypermobile joints often need neuromuscular reeducation, activating some muscle groups and addressing other dominant, tense muscles. For example, knee hypermobility is usually accompanied by quadriceps weakness and hamstring tightness. Exercising the quads and stretching the hamstrings helps to provide better muscular balance and control, often lessening the pain. Therapists should be free to address other compensatory mechanisms that are evident, such as lumbar hyperlordosis, which often accompanies the tight hamstrings, and/or flexible flat foot, which often loads the knee asymmetrically. Instruction and exercises to maintain proper posture and ergonomics are helpful, and repetitive activities, including activities of daily living, also often need to be addressed. A home exercise plan is important for long-term management and may include almost any desired physical activity, such as dancing or playing a sport.

Bracing and orthotics may play a role in joint support or protection and are used in conjunction with the therapy programs. Prolonged bracing may predispose to muscular weakness and atrophy if not paired with ongoing exercise but may be necessary, and is appropriate if used to enable routine activity, in the setting of injury, or when excessive strain is to be applied. Shoe orthotics are commonly ordered for flexible flat feet with heel valgus (**Fig. 2**). Somewhat characteristic for the hypermobility syndromes is laxity of the metacarpophalangeal and interphalangeal joints, for which digital ring splints are often helpful.

CHRONIC DIFFUSE PAIN

Pain is one of the top complaints of those with GJH, especially those with hEDS and HSD. Joint pain is particularly common in the load-bearing joints (ankles, knees, hips), joints involved in repetitive tasks (shoulders, wrists, and hands), as well as the back, neck, and the temporomandibular joints. Pain is often muscular with tender myotendinous insertion points and muscle tension with or without spasm. This condition may lead to chronic myofascial pain. The chronic pain can also lead to pain amplification or central sensitization, often diagnosed as fibromyalgia.[28,29] In addition to this nociceptive and central pain sensitization, neuropathic pain is also common.[26] Pain management is similar to other causes of pain, and includes physical therapy

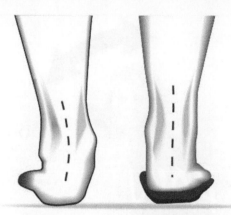

Fig. 2. Flexible pes planus with heel valgus. Heel valgus and proper biomechanics are restored using a shoe orthotic. (*Courtesy of* B.T. Tinkle, MD, PhD, Indianapolis, IN.)

(discussed earlier), medications, and psychological approaches (especially cognitive behavior therapy).[26,29]

HEADACHES

Headaches are one of the most debilitating and commonly encountered pains.[30–32] Headaches may be of multiple types, such as migraine,[30] daily persistent headache,[33] cervicogenic, temporomandibular joint dysfunction, or related to medications.[34] As with other types of pain, headache treatment is symptomatic and directed to the underlying causes.

FATIGUE

Many hypermobile people also complain of fatigue.[32,35] It is often both a mental and physical fatigue.[36] Joint pain and dysfunction can lead to physical deconditioning and worsen muscular endurance, causing more physical fatigue. Deconditioning can also exacerbate pain associated with routine daily activities, which can interfere with sleep. Sleep is often affected by a multitude of other factors, including anxiety, depression, dysautonomia, pain, and medications, all of which further contribute to fatigue and can cause a chronic cycle of pain and sleep disturbance (**Fig. 3**). This effective sleep deprivation can also result in both physical and mental fatigue. Dysautonomia is also common, manifesting as low blood pressure and postural dizziness with cyclical adrenaline surges to compensate for postural changes. This condition is speculated to interfere with the typical sleep cycle and many patients report temperature instability, restless sleep, or vivid dreaming.[37,38]

POSTURAL DIZZINESS

Postural dizziness (ie, orthostasis) with near syncope or frank syncope is also commonly encountered in this population, peaking in adolescence and young adulthood. Many show low blood pressure, particularly diastolic pressures in the 50s or low 60s (mm Hg). Studies in the general population suggest hypovolemia is a critical factor in adolescent girls. Inadequate fluid and salt intake are part of the problem, but other contributing factors could include anemia and/or menorrhagia. Those with joint hypermobility are even more susceptible to such orthostatic intolerance, although the

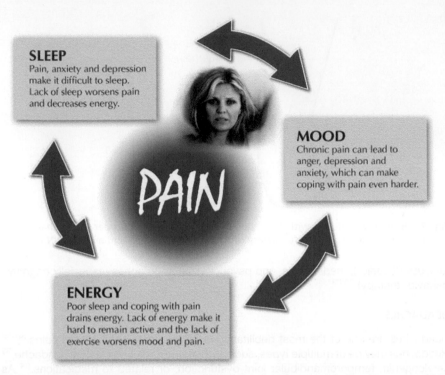

SLEEP
Pain, anxiety and depression make it difficult to sleep. Lack of sleep worsens pain and decreases energy.

MOOD
Chronic pain can lead to anger, depression and anxiety, which can make coping with pain even harder.

PAIN

ENERGY
Poor sleep and coping with pain drains energy. Lack of energy make it hard to remain active and the lack of exercise worsens mood and pain.

Fig. 3. Chronic pain cycle with effects on sleep, mood, and energy/vitality. (*Courtesy of* B.T. Tinkle, MD, PhD, Indianapolis, IN.)

underlying cause is not understood. Diagnostic testing may reveal postural orthostatic tachycardia syndrome, neutrally mediated hypotension, idiopathic supraventricular tachycardia, or simply orthostatic intolerance.[39] Of particular note is that hot showers and associated fainting have resulted in many patients with concussions (personal observation). Management includes aggressive hydration with increased sodium intake, compression garments, and avoidance of various triggers, such as heat and dehydration. Regular exercise may improve vascular tone, and treatment of menorrhagia or anemia as indicated is also helpful. Many patients do not require medications, but these may be helpful in select cases.[39] β-Blockers, fludrocortisone, and midodrine are the most commonly used pharmacologic treatments.

GASTROINTESTINAL

One of the earliest symptoms in those with systemic complications is often constipation. It is typically indistinct from chronic constipation of childhood and should be treated as such. However, as patients develop additional systemic manifestations, dysphagia, reflux, abdominal pain, bloating and/or diarrhea may be encountered. Gastroparesis occurs occasionally, but functional abdominal disorders still dominate.[40] Treatment follows similar avenues to patients without joint hypermobility. Nutritional approaches such as gluten-free or low-FODMAP (fermentable oligosaccharides, disaccharides, monosaccharides, and polyols) diets are the most common, along with hydration, exercise, proper toileting behaviors, and pelvic floor therapy as warranted.

SUMMARY

Joint hypermobility is easily evaluated using the Beighton scoring system in a clinical setting. It may portend joint laxity or instability that can put the patient at risk for mechanical injury but may also be asymptomatic. Joint hypermobility is often compensated for by muscular spasm, which can result in tension, pain, and fibromyalgia-like symptoms. It often responds well to physical therapy.

Those with more GJH may have further mechanical issues involving multiple, but not necessarily hypermobile, joints. GJH may also be a feature of a systemic disorder such as Marfan syndrome or one of the EDSs. Connective tissue abnormalities can involve the cardiovascular and gastrointestinal systems as well as the skin. Systemic manifestations may be many and may be subtle (such as low blood pressure) or may be symptomatic (such as orthostatic intolerance and syncope). Functional bowel disorders are also common. More generalized manifestations may be chronic pain or fatigue. These manifestations may be accompanied by sleep disturbance, poorer quality of life, as well as emotional and psychological issues such as anxiety or depressed mood. Such features are readily evaluated in a primary clinical setting and typically respond to standard treatment modalities. Other systemic complaints also follow similar management as in the general population. Objective, evidence-based interventional trials in those with GJH are scarce and much research is still needed.

REFERENCES

1. Castori M, Tinkle B, Levy H, et al. A framework for the classification of joint hypermobility and related conditions. Am J Med Genet C Semin Med Genet 2017; 175C:148–57. Available at: https://onlinelibrary.wiley.com/doi/epdf/10.1002/ajmg.c.31539.

2. Remvig L, Jensen DV, Ward RC. Epidemiology of general joint hypermobility and basis for the proposed criteria for benign joint hypermobility syndrome: review of the literature. J Rheumatol 2007;34:804–9.

3. Juul-Kristensen B, Schmedling K, Rombaut L, et al. Measurement properties of clinical assessment methods for classifying generalized joint hypermobility— A systematic review. Am J Med Genet Part C Semin Med Genet 2017;175C:116–47. Available at: https://onlinelibrary.wiley.com/doi/epdf/10.1002/ajmg.c.31540.

4. Beighton P, Solomon L, Soskolne CL. Articular mobility in an African population. Ann Rheum Dis 1973;32:413–8.

5. Remvig L, Jensen DV, Ward RC. Are diagnostic criteria for general joint hypermobility and benign joint hypermobility syndrome based on reproducible and valid tests? A review of the literature. J Rheumatol 2007;34:798–803.

6. Remvig L, Engelbert RH, Berglund B, et al. Need for a consensus on the methods by which to measure joint mobility and the definition of norms for hypermobility that reflect age, gender and ethnic-dependent variation: Is revision of criteria for joint hypermobility syndrome and Ehlers–Danlos syndrome hypermobility type indicated? Rheumatology 2011;50:1169–71.

7. Singh H, McKay M, Baldwin J, et al. Beighton scores and cut-offs across the lifespan: cross-sectional study of an Australian population. Rheumatology 2017;56: 1857–64.

8. Malfait F, Francomano C, Byers P, et al. The 2017 international classification of the Ehlers–Danlos syndromes. Am J Med Genet Part C Semin Med Genet 2017;175C: 8–26. Available at: https://onlinelibrary.wiley.com/doi/epdf/10.1002/ajmg.c.31552.

9. Grahame R, Bird HA, Child A, et al. The revised (Brighton 1998) criteria for the diagnosis of benign joint hypermobility syndrome (BJHS). J Rheumatol 2000; 27(7):1777–9.

10. Quatman CE, Ford KR, Myer GD, et al. The effects of gender and pubertal status on generalized joint laxity in young athletes. J Sci Med Sport 2008;11:257–63.

11. Castori M, Camerota F, Celletti C, et al. Ehlers–Danlos syndrome hypermobility type and the excess of affected females: Possible mechanisms and perspectives. Am J Med Genet A 2010;152A:2406–8.

12. Di Mattia F, Fary R, Murray KJ, et al. Two subtypes of symptomatic joint hypermobility: a descriptive study using latent class analysis. Arch Dis Child 2018 [pii:archdischild-2017-314149].

13. Hudson N, Fitzcharles MA, Cohen M, et al. The association of soft-tissue rheumatism and hypermobility. Br J Rheumatol 1998;37:382–6.

14. Cowderoy GA, Lisle DA, O'Connell PT. Overuse and impingement syndromes of the shoulder in the athlete. Magn Reason Imaging Clin N Am 2009;17:577–93.

15. Gupton M, Terreberry RR. Anatomy, hinge joints. In: StatPearls [Internet]. Treasure Island (FL): StatPearls Publishing; 2018. Available at: https://www.ncbi.nlm.nih.gov/books/NBK518967/. Accessed March 10, 2019.

16. Al-Rawi Z, Nessan AH. Joint hypermobility in patients with chondromalacia patellae. Br J Rheumatol 1997;36:1324–7.

17. Svoboda Z, Honzikova L, Janura M, et al. Kinematic gait analysis in children with valgus deformity of the hindfoot. Acta Bioeng Biomech 2014;16:89–93.

18. Kothari A, Dixon PC, Stebbins J, et al. Are flexible flat feet associated with proximal joint problems in children? Gait Posture 2016;45:204–10.

19. Noormohammadpour P, Borghei A, Mirzaei S, et al. The risk factors of low back pain in female high-school students. Spine (Phila Pa 1976) 2019;44(6):E357–65.

20. Online Mendelian Inheritance in Man, OMIM®. Baltimore (MD): McKusick-Nathans Institute of Genetic Medicine, Johns Hopkins University. Available at: https://omim.org/. Accessed March 10, 2019.

21. Bloom L, Byers P, Francomano C, et al. The international consortium on the Ehlers–Danlos syndromes. Am J Med Genet Part C Semin Med Genet 2017; 175C:5–7.

22. Kirk JA, Ansell BM, Bywaters EGL. The hypermobility syndrome. Musculoskeletal complaints associated with generalized joint hypermobility. Ann Rheum Dis 1967; 26:419–25.

23. Beighton P, De Paepe A, Steinmann B, et al. Ehlers-Danlos syndromes: revised nosology, Villefranche, 1997. Ehlers-Danlos National Foundation (USA) and Ehlers-Danlos Support Group (UK). Am J Med Genet 1998;77:31–7.

24. Tinkle BT, Bird HA, Grahame R, et al. The lack of clinical distinction between the hypermobility type of Ehlers-Danlos syndrome and the joint hypermobility syndrome (a.k.a. hypermobility syndrome). Am J Med Genet A 2009;149A:2368–70.

25. Castori M, Morlino S, Celletti C, et al. Re-writing the natural history of pain and related symptoms in the joint hypermobility syndrome/Ehlers-Danlos syndrome, hypermobility type. Am J Med Genet Part A 2013;161A:2989–3004.

26. Tinkle B, Castori M, Berglund B, et al. Hypermobile Ehlers–Danlos syndrome (a.k.a. Ehlers–Danlos syndrome Type III and Ehlers–Danlos syndrome hypermobility type): clinical description and natural history. Am J Med Genet Part C Semin Med Genet 2017;175C:48–69. Available at: https://onlinelibrary.wiley.com/doi/epdf/10.1002/ajmg.c.31538.

27. Engelbert RH, Juul-Kristensen B, Pacey V, et al. The evidence-based rationale for physical therapy treatment of children, adolescents, and adults diagnosed with

joint hypermobility syndrome/hypermobile Ehlers Danlos syndrome. Am J Med Genet Part C Semin Med Genet 2017;175C:158–67. Available at: https://onlinelibrary.wiley.com/doi/epdf/10.1002/ajmg.c.31545.

28. Ting TV, Hashkes PJ, Schikler K, et al. The role of benign joint hypermobility in the pain experience in juvenile fibromyalgia: an observational study. Pediatr Rheumatol Online J 2012;10:16.

29. Chopra P, Tinkle B, Hamonet C, et al. Pain management in the Ehlers–Danlos syndromes. Am J Med Genet Part C Semin Med Genet 2017;175C:212–9. Available at: https://onlinelibrary.wiley.com/doi/epdf/10.1002/ajmg.c.31554.

30. Bendik EM, Tinkle BT, Al-shuik E, et al. Joint hypermobility syndrome: a common clinical disorder associated with migraine in women. Cephalalgia 2011;31: 603–13.

31. Jacome DE. Headache in Ehlers-Danlos syndrome. Cephalalgia 1999;19:791–6.

32. Murray B, Yashar BM, Uhlmann WR, et al. Ehlers-Danlos syndrome, hypermobility type: a characterization of the patients' lived experience. Am J Med Genet Part A 2013;161A:2981–8.

33. Rozen TD, Roth JM, Denenberg N. Joint hypermobility as a predisposing factor for the development of new daily persistent headache. Headache 2005;45: 828–9.

34. Neilson D, Martin VT. Joint hypermobility and headache: understanding the glue that binds the two together- part 1. Headache 2014;54:1393–402.

35. Voermans NC, Knoop H, van de Kamp N, et al. Fatigue is a frequent and clinically relevant problem in Ehlers-Danlos syndrome. Semin Arthritis Rheum 2010;40: 267–74.

36. Rowe PC, Barron DF, Calkins H, et al. Orthostatic intolerance and chronic fatigue syndrome associated with Ehlers-Danlos syndrome. J Pediatr 1999;135:494–9.

37. Kizilbash SJ, Ahrens SP, Bruce BK, et al. Adolescent fatigue, POTS, and recovery: a guide for clinicians. Curr Probl Pediatr Adolesc Health Care 2014;44: 108–33.

38. Hakim A, De Wandele I, O'Callaghan C, et al. Chronic fatigue in Ehlers–Danlos syndrome—hypermobile type. Am J Med Genet Part C Semin Med Genet 2017;175C:175–80. Available at: https://onlinelibrary.wiley.com/doi/epdf/10.1002/ajmg.c.31542.

39. Hakim A, O'Callaghan C, De Wandele I, et al. Cardiovascular autonomic dysfunction in Ehlers–Danlos syndrome—Hypermobile type. Am J Med Genet Part C Semin Med Genet 2017;175C:168–74. Available at: https://onlinelibrary.wiley.com/doi/epdf/10.1002/ajmg.c.31543.

40. Fikree A, Chelimsky G, Collins H, et al. Gastrointestinal involvement in the Ehlers–Danlos syndromes. Am J Med Genet Part C Semin Med Genet 2017;175C:181–7. Available at: https://onlinelibrary.wiley.com/doi/epdf/10.1002/ajmg.c.31546.

The Diagnosis and Management of Neurofibromatosis Type 1

K. Ina Ly, MD[a],*, Jaishri O. Blakeley, MD[b,c]

KEYWORDS

- Neurofibromatosis type 1 • Tumor predisposition syndrome • Nervous system
- RASopathy • Plexiform neurofibroma • Cutaneous neurofibroma

KEY POINTS

- The neurofibromatoses (neurofibromatosis type 1 [NF1], neurofibromatosis type 2, and schwannomatosis) are related, but distinct, autosomal dominant tumor predisposition conditions characterized by tumors in the central and peripheral nervous systems. NF1 is the most common, with an estimated prevalence of 1 in 3000.
- NF1 has phenotypic overlap with other RASopathies, a group of rare genetic conditions caused by mutations in the Ras/mitogen-activated protein kinase pathway.
- Clinical diagnostic criteria for NF1 are sensitive across the lifespan. However, variability in presentation can complicate clinical diagnosis, particularly in early childhood. Molecular testing is highly sensitive and specific.
- Multidisciplinary care is necessary for patients with NF1, given the range of severity and type of manifestations inherent in the condition.

INTRODUCTION

Neurofibromatosis (NF) type 1 (NF1), NF type 2 (NF2), and schwannomatosis constitute a group of autosomal dominant tumor suppressor syndromes that predispose to benign and malignant tumors. Although there is a predilection for involvement of the nervous system, the NFs, particularly NF1, involve a spectrum of organ systems.

Disclosures: Dr K.I. Ly has nothing to disclose. Dr J.O. Blakeley receives research support from GlaxoSmithKline and served as a paid consultant for Abbvie and an unpaid consultant for Astra Zenica, Exelixis, and Springworks Therapeutics. She has served as the study principal investigator for clinical trials supported by Sanofi-Aventis and by Lily.

[a] Stephen E. and Catherine Pappas Center for Neuro-Oncology, Massachusetts General Hospital, Yawkey 9 East, 55 Fruit Street, Boston, MA 02114, USA; [b] Department of Neurology and Neurosurgery, Johns Hopkins University, 600 North Wolfe Street, Meyer 100, Baltimore, MD 21287, USA; [c] Department of Oncology, Johns Hopkins University, 600 North Wolfe Street, Meyer 100, Baltimore, MD 21287, USA
* Corresponding author.
E-mail address: ily@partners.org

Med Clin N Am 103 (2019) 1035–1054
https://doi.org/10.1016/j.mcna.2019.07.004
0025-7125/19/© 2019 Elsevier Inc. All rights reserved.

NF1 is the most common form of NF (estimated birth incidence of 1 in 2500 and prevalence of 1 in 2000 to 1 in 4000) and one of the most common autosomal dominant diseases of the nervous system.[1–3] Hallmark cutaneous findings include café-au-lait macules (CALMs), skinfold freckling, and cutaneous neurofibromas (cNFs) (**Figs. 1 and 2**). Some of these cutaneous features can also be seen in NF2 and other related conditions (RASopathies) that involve dysregulation of the Ras/mitogen-activated protein kinase (MAPK) signaling pathway.[4] Among these disorders, NF1 carries the highest malignancy risk (estimated lifetime cancer risk, 59.6%).[5] Hence, it is critical to accurately identify individuals with NF1 to optimize clinical management, genetic counseling, and malignancy surveillance.

This article focuses on the clinical characteristics, diagnostic evaluation, and management of NF1. A brief overview of NF2, schwannomatosis, and related syndromes and the features that distinguish them from NF1 is included (**Table 1** and **2**).

Epidemiology

NF1 is an autosomal dominant condition but the estimated new mutation rate is unusually high. Approximately 42% of affected individuals have de novo mutations rather than inheriting it from an affected parent.[1] All ethnicities, races, and sexes are affected with equal frequency.[6]

Diagnostic Criteria

The National Institutes of Health (NIH) clinical diagnostic criteria for NF1[7,8] (**Table 2**) are highly specific and sensitive in most patients except very young individuals and those with mosaic involvement or with variants lacking characteristic skin findings.[9] Approximately 46% of patients with sporadic NF1 (ie, de novo mutations) do not meet criteria by age 1 year. If NF1 is suspected, annual monitoring until late childhood is necessary because 97% of children with at least 1 feature of NF1 eventually meet diagnostic criteria by age 8 years.[10]

Differential Diagnosis

NF1 may clinically overlap with other types of NF and other conditions such as Legius syndrome, constitutional mismatch repair deficiency syndrome,[11] and Noonan syndrome[12] (see **Table 1**).

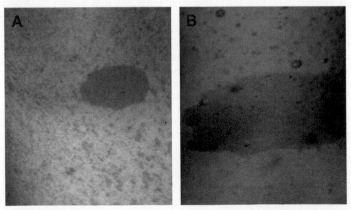

Fig. 1. (A) Café-au-lait macule in a region of axillary freckling. (B) Café-au-lait macule with cutaneous neurofibromas.

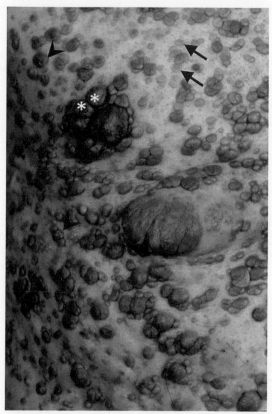

Fig. 2. Heterogeneous morphologic appearance of cutaneous neurofibromas in a single patient, including sessile (*arrows*), globular (*arrowheads*), and pedunculated (*asterisks*) cNFs. (*From* Ortonne N, Wolkenstein P, Blakeley JO, et al. Cutaneous neurofibromas: Current clinical and pathologic issues. Neurology 2018;91(2 Supplement 1):S8; with permission.)

- NF2 is approximately 10 times less common than NF1 (estimated incidence, 1 in 30000).[13,14] More than 95% of patients with NF2 have bilateral vestibular schwannomas.[14] Other characteristic tumors are schwannomas of the nonvestibular cranial, spinal, and peripheral nerves; meningiomas (often multiple); and spinal cord ependymomas (see **Tables 1** and **2**).[7,15] NF2-associated schwannomas are highly unlikely to become malignant. Schwannomas can also manifest in the skin as intracutaneous plaquelike lesions or deep-seated subcutaneous nodules; CALMs are rare.[16,17] Typical ocular manifestations are cataracts, retinal hamartomas, epiretinal membranes, and optic nerve meningiomas.[16,18] NF2 does not predispose to cognitive impairment.
- Schwannomatosis (estimated incidence, 1 in 69000)[14] is characterized by multiple schwannomas, most commonly affecting the spinal (74%) and peripheral nerves (89%); cranial nerve schwannomas (8%) and meningiomas (5%) are rare (see **Tables 1** and **2**).[19–22] Skin manifestations are limited to schwannomas, and there are no known ocular features.
- Legius syndrome is found in approximately 2% of people meeting NIH diagnostic criteria for NF1.[23] This condition causes CALMs with or without skinfold freckling and sometimes learning disabilities, but not neurofibromas, Lisch nodules,

Table 1
Clinical features of neurofibromatoses and related disorders

Disease	Genes	Inheritance	Tumors	Cutaneous Features	Ocular Features
NF1	*NF1* (germline)	AD	• Neurofibroma (cutaneous, plexiform)[a] • OPG • MPNST • GIST • Pheochromocytoma • Breast cancer • JMML	• CALMs • Skinfold freckling • Cutaneous neurofibromas	• Lisch nodules • OPG
Segmental NF1	*NF1* (postzygotic, somatic)	Somatic mutation but may lead to AD inheritance	• Neurofibroma (cutaneous, plexiform)[a,b] • OPG[a,b]	• CALMs[b] • Skinfold freckling[b] • Cutaneous neurofibromas[a]	• Lisch nodules (rare)
NF2	*NF2*	AD	• Bilateral vestibular schwannoma[a] • Meningioma (~80% by age 70 y) • Spinal ependymoma	• Cutaneous or intradermal schwannomas • CALMs (rare)	• Cataracts (posterior subcapsular lenticular opacities) • Retinal hamartomas • Epiretinal membranes • Optic nerve meningioma
Schwannomatosis	*SMARCB1, LZTR1*	AD	• Schwannoma[a] • Meningioma (rare)	• Subcutaneous schwannomas	None known
Legius syndrome	*SPRED1*	AD	None	• CALMs • Skinfold freckling	None known

CMMRD	MLH1, MSH2, MSH6, PMS2	AR	• Hematologic cancers (predominance of T-cell non-Hodgkin lymphoma) • Malignant gliomas (eg, glioblastomas) • Colorectal and other cancers associated with Lynch syndrome • Sarcomas, embryonic tumors (rare) • Note: higher risk of malignancy than NF1	• CALMs • Skinfold freckling (rare)	• Lisch nodules (very rare) • OPG (very rare)
Noonan syndrome	PTPN11 (~50%), other genes in RAS-MAPK pathway	AD	• Hematologic cancers • Embryonic tumors (rare)	• CALMs	• Strabismus, refractive errors, amblyopia, nystagmus • Cataracts • Fundal changes

Abbreviations: AD, autosomal dominant; AR, autosomal recessive; CMMRD, constitutional mismatch repair deficiency syndrome; GIST, gastrointestinal stromal tumor; JMML, juvenile myelomonocytic leukemia; MPNST, malignant peripheral nerve sheath tumor; OPG, optic pathway glioma.

[a] Hallmark tumor.

[b] occurring in only a portion of the body.

Table 2
Clinical diagnostic criteria for neurofibromatosis type 1, neurofibromatosis type 2, and schwannomatosis

NF1[7,8]	NF2[7,15]	Schwannomatosis[20–22]
Presence of ≥2 of the following: 1. ≥6 CALMs >5 mm in diameter in prepubertal individuals and >15 mm in postpubertal individuals 2. ≥2 neurofibromas of any type or 1 plexiform neurofibroma 3. Freckling in the axillary or inguinal regions 4. ≥2 Lisch nodules 5. Optic glioma 6. A distinctive osseous lesion such as sphenoid wing dysplasia or thinning of long bone cortex, with or without pseudoarthrosis 7. First-degree relative (parents, sibling, or offspring) with NF1 based on above criteria	Any 1 of the following: 1. Bilateral VS before age 70 y 2. Unilateral VS before age 70 y and first-degree relative with NF2 3. Any 2 of the following: meningioma, nonvestibular schwannoma, neurofibroma, glioma, cerebral calcification, cataract, and • First-degree relative with NF2, or • Unilateral VS and negative *LZTR1* testing[a] 4. Multiple meningiomas and • Unilateral VS or • Any 2 of the following: nonvestibular schwannoma, neurofibroma, glioma, cerebral calcification, cataract 5. Constitutional or mosaic pathogenic *NF2* mutation from blood or by identification of an identical mutation from 2 separate tumors in the same individual	Definite Age>30 y and all of the following: • ≥2 nonintradermal schwannomas (at least 1 with histologic confirmation) • Diagnostic criteria for NF2 not fulfilled • No evidence of vestibular tumor on high-quality MRI scan • No first-degree relative with NF2 • No known constitutional *NF2* mutation Or Age>30 y and 1 pathologically confirmed nonvestibular schwannoma and a first-degree relative who meets above criteria Possible Age<30 y and all the following: • ≥2 nonintradermal schwannomas (at least 1 with histologic confirmation) • Diagnostic criteria for NF2 not fulfilled • No evidence of vestibular tumor on high-quality MRI scan • No first-degree relative with NF2 • No known constitutional *NF2* mutation Or Age>45 y and all of the following: • ≥2 nonintradermal schwannomas (at least 1 with histologic confirmation) • No symptoms of eighth cranial nerve dysfunction • No first-degree relative with NF2 • No known constitutional *NF2* mutation Or Radiographic evidence of a nonvestibular schwannoma and first-degree relative meeting criteria for definite schwannomatosis

Note that children of a parent with known NF1 are often diagnosed with NF1 by age 1 year because they already meet 1 criterion (having a first-degree relative with NF1). Their second criterion is commonly CALMs, which, although not specific for NF1, is often present at birth.

Abbreviation: VS, vestibular schwannoma.

[a] If qualifying tumors include greater than or equal to 2 nonintradermal schwannomas.

symptomatic optic pathway gliomas, or osseous lesions (see **Table 1**).[23,24] Legius syndrome and NF1 cannot be distinguished based on CALMs and freckling alone, and genetic testing is recommended.

Genetics, Molecular Pathophysiology, and Genotype-Phenotype Correlations

NF1 occurs as a result of a germline mutation in one of the 2 alleles of the tumor suppressor gene *NF1* on chromosome 17q11.2.[25,26] Although this heterozygous germline mutation is sufficient to cause NF1, somatic loss of function in the second allele is required for tumor formation. The protein product, neurofibromin, is important in regulating Ras, a proto-oncogene that plays a prominent role in cell growth and differentiation and is mutated in many common cancers.[27] Neurofibromin is expressed in most tissues but at particularly high levels in the nervous system (including Schwann cells along peripheral nerve trunks, glial cells, and neurons),[28] which partially explains the predilection for peripheral nerve sheath tumors and gliomas.

Mosaic NF1 occurs when there is a somatic mutation later in embryonic development (as opposed to a germline mutation in generalized NF1). Mutations that occur very early in embryonic development can present with a phenotype similar to generalized NF1, whereas mutations in terminally differentiated cells typically manifest with isolated areas of involvement.[29] Clinically, the area of involvement may vary from a narrow strip to one-half of the body; although often unilateral, it sometimes involves both sides.[29] The rate of transmission of *NF1* mutations to the offspring of those with mosaic NF1 ranges from 0% to 50% (depending on the degree to which the gonads are affected by the *NF1* mutation).[14] In individuals with suspected mosaic NF1, genetic testing should be performed on blood as well as on the affected tissue (eg, melanocytes from a CALM).[30]

The type and severity of NF1 clinical manifestations are highly variable between individuals, including among members of the same family.[31] Although more than 2800 different pathogenic variants have been identified in the *NF1* gene, only 31 are common enough to be found in more than a few affected individuals.[32] However, some genotype-phenotype correlations are emerging. *NF1* gene microdeletions[33] and mutations of certain *NF1* codons[32] typically confer a more severe phenotype, whereas other mutations and small deletions are associated with a phenotype limited to CALMs and freckling, milder cognitive impairment, and/or lower risk of neoplasms (**Box 1**).[34–38] Knowledge about these genotype-phenotype correlations can provide prognostic guidance and aid in organ-specific surveillance. Therefore, although genetic testing has historically been reserved for equivocal diagnostic cases, these genotype-phenotype relationships lead to increasing demand to pursue genetic testing to understand the type of pathogenic mutation and permit more precise interventions.

Clinical Features, Diagnostic Evaluation, and Management

Café-au-lait macules

CALMs are frequently the first presenting sign of NF1: 99% have 6 or more CALMs by age 1 year[10,39] and greater than or equal to 75% of individuals with 6 or more CALMs eventually meet diagnostic criteria for NF1.[40,41] CALMs usually increase in number during early childhood, stabilizing or even fading over time (**Tables 3 and 4**). Typical CALMs are flat, uniformly hyperpigmented macules with regular, well-defined borders (see **Fig. 1**).[40] Atypical CALMs have irregular borders and inhomogeneous pigmentation[42] and are less likely to be associated with NF1 than typical CALMs.[40] Although CALM morphology may be a useful predictor of

---

Box 1
Indications for genetic testing

To diagnose variant forms of NF1 or diagnose young children who do not yet meet clinical diagnostic criteria

To confirm suspected mosaic NF1: need to include affected tissue and blood for testing

To establish genotype-phenotype correlations
  More severe phenotype:
  • *NF1* gene microdeletions: large numbers of neurofibromas, facial dysmorphism, developmental delay, intellectual disability, increased risk for malignant peripheral nerve sheath tumors
  • Missense mutation of codons 844 to 848: optic pathway gliomas (OPGs), superficial plexiform neurofibromas, symptomatic spinal neurofibromas, skeletal abnormalities, higher risk of malignancy
  Milder phenotypes:
  • Single amino acid deletion at position 2971: CALMs, freckling
  • Missense mutations at codon Arg 1809: developmental delay, learning disability, pulmonic stenosis, Noonan-like features, no superficial plexiform neurofibromas or symptomatic OPGs
  • In-frame deletion of 3 bp of exon 17 (c2970_2972del p.Met992del): pigmentary changes, cognitive manifestations possible, no cutaneous or superficial plexiform neurofibromas

To differentiate between NF1 and other RASopathies; for example:
• Legius syndrome
• Constitutional mismatch repair deficiency syndrome
• Noonan syndrome

Preimplantation and prenatal genetic testing (if desired by parents)

In general, this should be considered in individuals with an unclear clinical diagnosis or in whom a definitive molecular diagnosis can guide surveillance relative to the organ systems most likely to be affected and aid in prognosis.

---

the presence or absence of NF1, it is subject to significant interrater variability, so all children with ≥6 CALMs (whether typical or atypical) should be referred for specialist evaluation. Some clinicians suggest referral for patients with ≥ 3 CALMs, given the low incidence of ≥3 CALMs in the general population without an associated systemic disorder.[40] In children younger than 8 years, if the only clinical finding is ≥ three CALMs, surveillance during routine pediatric evaluations for other NF1 manifestations is likely sufficient.[43] Evaluation for CALMs ideally involves comprehensive skin examination under ambient light and, if difficult to detect, a Wood lamp (a device that emits long-wave ultraviolet light used in a darkened room). The latter may be particularly useful in individuals with dark skin tones.

Freckling
Skinfold freckling occurs in up to 90% of patients by age 7 years.[10,39] Freckles are smaller than CALMs and typically involve areas of skin apposition, particularly the axillary and inguinal regions, but can also involve other intertriginous areas such as the neckline or inframammary region in women.[39] Some patients develop more diffuse freckling (see **Fig. 1**).

Cutaneous neurofibromas
Cutaneous neurofibromas (cNFs), the most common tumor in NF1, are seen in greater than 99% of adult patients (see **Fig. 2**).[44] These slow-growing lesions involve the epidermis and dermis, present in late childhood, and increase in number with age.[39]

Table 3
Recommended diagnostic evaluation and management strategies for common clinical features of neurofibromatosis type 1. Guidelines for the care of adults and children with neurofibromatosis type 1 were recently published by the American College of Medical Genetics and Genomics[61] and the American Academy of Pediatrics[95]

Feature	Diagnostic Evaluation	Management
CALMs and skinfold freckling	• Skin examination • Referral to genetics, NF specialist or dermatologists if >6 CALMs	• None required • Consider dermatologic camouflage treatment if cosmetically distressing
Cutaneous neurofibromas	• Skin examination • Referral to genetics, NF specialist or dermatologist	• If symptomatic (eg, painful or pruritic) or disfiguring, refer to dermatologist or plastic surgeon for electrodessication, CO_2 laser treatment, or surgical removal or consideration of clinical trial
Lisch nodules	• Referral to (neuro)-ophthalmologist for slit-lamp examination to help establish or confirm diagnosis of NF1	• No monitoring or treatment needed
Plexiform neurofibromas	• Annual physical and neurologic examination • Regional MRI (with contrast) of symptomatic body part • Possibly whole-body MRI surveillance	• Repeat MRI for surveillance if moderate or high risk for progression or malignant transformation including if the patient reports worsening symptoms (eg, pain, loss of function of body part, cosmetically disturbing) • Referral to neurosurgery, or orthopedic or plastic surgeon for resection of symptomatic lesions • Consideration of drug therapy via clinical trials; management of symptoms including pain management
MPNST	• Regional MRI (with contrast) of symptomatic body part for anatomic delineation • PET imaging to confirm malignancy and identify "hot spots" to guide biopsy • Referral to surgeon for biopsy ± resection and histologic confirmation	• Multidisciplinary management is required from initial suspicion of cancer diagnosis to allow for appropriate sequencing of therapies including chemotherapy, radiation therapy, surgery and clinical trials

(continued on next page)

Table 3
(continued)

Feature	Diagnostic Evaluation	Management
	• Referral to radiation oncologist and sarcoma specialist	
OPGs	• Referral to (neuro)-ophthalmologist for eye examination to be done annually for all people <10 y old and in some practices through adulthood • MRI of orbits and brain if eye examination is abnormal • Annual height and weight measurement to screen for precocious puberty	• Consider continued annual ophthalmologic screening through adulthood or for 10–25 y after initial diagnosis of OPG • Referral to NF specialist or oncologist for management based on MRI and ophthalmologic examination findings
Behavioral/learning difficulties	• Referral to psychologist for neurocognitive testing • Referral to psychiatrist	• Academic support, including individualized educational plan, and physical, occupational, and speech therapy • Consider pharmacologic management of behavioral difficulties
Scoliosis, long bone pseudoarthrosis	• Plain radiographs	• Referral to orthopedic surgeon for consideration of bracing ± surgery
Osteopenia/osteoporosis	• DEXA scan • Vitamin D level	• Calcium + vitamin D supplementation ± bisphosphonates • Regular follow-up DEXA scan
Hypertension	• Blood pressure measurement	• Routine blood pressure measurement, including during childhood • Consider work-up for secondary causes, especially in cases of severe hypertension and those refractory to pharmacologic treatment
Breast cancer	• Mammogram	• Annual mammogram starting at age 30 y • Aggressive management of breast cancers, including consideration of bilateral mastectomy after confirmed diagnosis of breast cancer

Abbreviation: DEXA, dual-energy X-ray absorptiometry.

Table 4
Typical timeline of appearance of cardinal features of neurofibromatosis type 1

Clinical Feature	Typical Time of Appearance
CALMs	Birth to age 2 y
Anterolateral tibial bowing/dysplasia (congenital lesions)	Infancy to age 5 y
Skinfold freckling	Age 3–8 y
Symptomatic optic pathway glioma	Age 0–10 y
Lisch nodules	Age 5–10 y
Scoliosis	• Dysplastic (rapidly progressive) form: age 6–10 y • Mild form: adolescence
Cutaneous neurofibromas	Mid to late childhood to early adulthood
Diffuse plexiform neurofibromas (congenital lesions)	• Tumors of face and neck: before age 1 y • Tumors of other body parts: before adolescence
MPNSTs	Adolescence or adulthood

In 1 study, 10% of people $\leq$ 10 years old had up to 10 cNFs, whereas >85% of people >40 years old had >100 cNFs.[45] cNFs should be distinguished from diffusely infiltrating plexiform neurofibromas (pNFs) that arise in deeper tissues and invade into the dermis.[46] This distinction is important because atypia seen on biopsy of cNF almost always reflects reactive or degenerative changes rather than malignant conversion, whereas similar atypia in pNFs infiltrating the skin could signal early malignant transformation.[47] cNFs seem to grow more rapidly during puberty and pregnancy, but prospective studies to address the factors associated with this observation are lacking.[44,48,49] Morphologically, cNFs can appear as nascent/latent, flat, sessile, globular, and pedunculated lesions[46] (see **Fig. 2**); it is unclear whether these categories represent evolutionary stages of cNFs or unique subtypes. cNFs range in size from 0.5 to 30 mm, are soft, and are generally nontender. Associated pruritus is reported in ~20% of patients.[50] Although cNF are histologically benign, they can cause significant disfigurement and emotional and physical discomfort, and directly contribute to decreased quality of life.[51]

The current mainstay of treatment of cNFs is physical removal, which is effective in many instances (see **Table 3**).[52] However, given that some patients have extensive skin involvement, it is often not feasible to remove all tumors, and multiple treatment sessions are frequently needed. Additional disadvantages of physical removal include the risk of scarring, regrowth of tumors, and appearance of new tumors over time.[52,53]

Lisch nodules
Lisch nodules typically appear between the ages of 5 and 10 years and are detected in more than 70% by age 10 years (see **Table 4**).[10,39] These nodules are well-defined, dome-shaped, melanocytic hamartomas of the iris. They are clear to yellow or brown, approximately 2 mm in size, and often visible with the naked eye. However, a slit-lamp examination is required to differentiate Lisch nodules from iris nevi, which are flat or minimally elevated pigmented lesions with blurred margins.[54] Lisch nodules do not impact vision nor do they have neoplastic potential. They are only present in 5% of children less than 3 years old with NF1, but prevalence increases with age such that most adults with NF1 have Lisch nodules.[54] All patients with suspected NF1 should be referred to an ophthalmologist for slit-lamp examination for potential Lisch nodules. An ophthalmology evaluation is also required to evaluate for signs

associated with optic pathway glioma in children and retinal vascular abnormalities in adults.[55]

Plexiform neurofibromas

Plexiform neurofibromas (pNFs) are histologically benign tumors of the peripheral nerve sheath affecting 40% to 50% of patients with NF1.[56,57] They may cause disfigurement and be visible to the naked eye or may be located deep inside the body. When asymptomatic, internal pNFs may only be detected with MRI. Regardless of location, pNFs can cause significant morbidity because of pain, disfigurement, local compression, and loss of function of nerves, great vessels, and airways.[58] They are also associated with increased mortality, given the risk of transformation into malignant peripheral nerve sheath tumors (MPNSTs). Any change in the severity and nature of symptoms (eg, interval growth, increased pain) should prompt evaluation for malignant transformation. Patients with new neurologic symptoms or signs (eg, focal limb weakness, sensory changes) should undergo MRI to evaluate for pNF. pNFs grow most rapidly during childhood and adolescence, followed by slowed or no growth thereafter.[59] Therefore, pNF growth in adulthood warrants close surveillance for possible malignant transformation.[56,59] MRI is the gold standard imaging modality to diagnose pNFs and may reveal heterogeneous growth patterns and radiographic appearances. Diffuse pNFs asymmetrically infiltrate peripheral nerves and do not have clear borders (**Fig. 3**A). Nodular pNFs are round/ovoid and have well demarcated margins (**Fig. 3**B, C).[60]

The current standard of care for pNFs is a comprehensive annual physical examination to detect symptomatic tumors. However, there are no recommendations on the frequency or type of surveillance imaging (eg, regional vs whole-body MRI).[43,61] In particular, it is unclear how often asymptomatic patients with known pNFs should be imaged. Some physicians obtain a baseline MRI of asymptomatic visible tumors, whereas others reserve imaging for symptomatic tumors only. Indications for surgical resection of pNFs are neurologic impairment, pain, and severe disfigurement, with the goal to restore or protect function. However, surgery is often challenging or not feasible because of involvement of nervous system structures. Promising medical therapies are currently under investigation, including selumetinib (a mitogen-activated

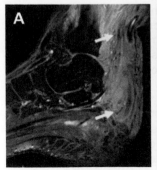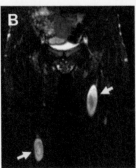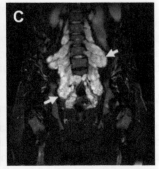

Fig. 3. Varying appearance of pNFs on MRI. (A) Sagittal T1-weighted postcontrast image of a diffusely infiltrating pNF of the left ankle (arrows), involving the skin, subcutaneous tissues, muscles, and intramuscular fascia. (B) Coronal short tau inversion recovery (STIR) image of 2 solitary nodular pNFs (arrows) involving the bilateral thighs. Note that the signal intensity appears more homogeneous than in MPNSTs (see **Fig. 4**). (C) Coronal STIR image of multiple pNFs arising from the lumbar and sacral foramina (arrows) and extending along the lumbosacral nerves.

protein kinase 1 (MEK) inhibitor), which has shown partial response rates of 72% in an interim analysis of a phase II trial.[62]

Malignant peripheral nerve sheath tumors

MPNSTs occur in 8% to 16% of patients with NF1[5] and are the leading cause of death in this population, with a 5-year survival rate of 15% to 50%.[63] Several clinical factors seem to be associated with MPNST development, including the number and volume of internal pNFs,[60,64,65] presence of subcutaneous neurofibromas,[60,65] younger age,[65] presence of pain,[66] NF1 gene microdeletion,[67] family/personal history of MPNST,[68] and presence of atypical neurofibromas.[47,69] MPNSTs most often develop within pre-existing pNFs,[47,70] but may also arise de novo. On MRI, they are typically associated with peripheral enhancement, peripheral edema, intratumoral cystic lesions, necrosis, and heterogeneous signal intensity[71] (**Fig. 4**), although there is some radiographic overlap between benign and malignant tumors.[72] Functional MRI and PET have high sensitivity for malignant transformation and may help identify the optimal site for biopsy.[73,74,75]

For localized disease, complete resection with wide negative margins is potentially curative. However, this is only feasible if the tumor is identified early and can be clearly defined and removed without significant neurologic and functional morbidity. Gross total resection and surgical margin status are important prognostic factors, independent of tumor size, grade, and provision of radiation.[76] Adjuvant radiation is sometimes provided to reduce the risk of local recurrence (particularly if wide surgical margins cannot be achieved) and as a limb-salvaging strategy. Adjuvant chemotherapy has a role in advanced or metastatic disease, but prognosis remains poor even with treatment.[63]

Optic pathway and other central nervous system gliomas

Optic pathway gliomas (OPGs) are the most common type of gliomas in NF1 and affect 15% to 20% of patients. However, only 30% to 50% develop symptoms and, of those, only one-third require intervention.[77] On histology, most OPGs are

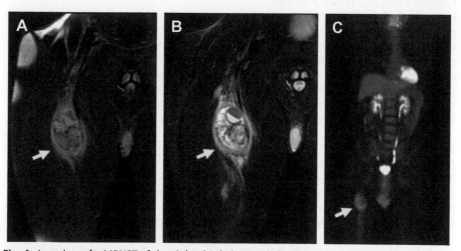

Fig. 4. Imaging of a MPNST of the right thigh (*arrows*). (*A, B*) Coronal T1-weighted postcontrast and STIR images show a mass lesion with heterogeneous signal intensity, reflecting a mixture of tumor cells, necrosis, edema, and cystic changes. (*C*) PET images reveal increased tracer uptake in this region, confirming the suspicion of malignant degeneration.

low-grade pilocytic astrocytomas.[77] They can arise anywhere along the optic pathway. Symptoms depend on tumor location and include proptosis, decreased visual acuity, visual field defect, precocious puberty (caused by hypothalamic involvement), and, rarely, symptoms of obstructive hydrocephalus such as headache, nausea, and vomiting.[77]

Given that most OPGs are asymptomatic and neither progress nor require treatment, the goal of surveillance is to detect symptomatic OPGs. Current guidelines recommend annual eye examinations for all patients less than 10 years old.[39,78] There is less consensus on screening frequency after age 10 years; some centers perform screening at least every 2 years until the age of 18 years or for 10 to 25 years after initial diagnosis.[78] Screening includes ophthalmologic evaluation of visual acuity, visual fields, and color vision, and anatomic evaluation of the eye.[77] If the eye examination is abnormal, MRI of the brain and orbits should be obtained. In addition, all children should undergo yearly height and weight measurements to screen for precocious puberty.[78]

The mainstay of treatment is chemotherapy with carboplatin (with or without vincristine), which stabilizes and potentially decreases tumor size. Notably, even with treatment, children rarely regain normal visual acuity.[77] Radiation is typically avoided because of the potential risk of vascular complications and secondary malignancies. In addition, young patients are at high risk of significant radiation-induced neurocognitive sequelae.[77] Additional therapies (such as selumetinib) are under investigation.

Other types of gliomas are much less common in NF1, although more common than in the general population. Brainstem lesions may represent gliomas and comprise approximately 18% of NF1-associated lesions,[79] but they tend to be less aggressive and more frequently found incidentally than their sporadic counterparts.[80] High-grade gliomas are rare in NF1 (<3% of patients with NF1 with central nervous system tumors).[81] However, the natural history of adult and pediatric gliomas suggests that otherwise benign histology can act more aggressively in adults with NF1.[82]

Cognitive and behavioral problems

Up to 81% of children with NF1 show moderate to severe impairment in ≥1 cognitive domain and almost 40% fulfill diagnostic criteria for attention-deficit/hyperactivity disorder.[83] The incidence of intellectual disability (full-scale intelligence quotient <70) is only slightly higher than in the general population, ranging from 4% to 8%.[84] All children with NF1 should be monitored closely for developmental delays and behavioral problems. Academic support should be provided early to those with learning disabilities, and then reassessed intermittently throughout the child's development. Children with attention-deficit/hyperactivity disorder may require stimulant medications.

Bone abnormalities

NF1-associated orthopedic problems present most commonly in early childhood and include scoliosis, osteopenia or osteoporosis, tibial dysplasia and pseudoarthrosis (a false joint caused by nonunion of a long bone fracture), and sphenoid wing dysplasia.[85,86] Scoliosis affects 21% to 49% of patients with NF1 and can be severe and progress more rapidly than in the general population.[85] Hence, children with NF1 should be evaluated regularly for scoliosis with examination and plain films and, if there are changes, referred to an orthopedic surgeon. Anterolateral tibial bowing and tibial dysplasia are congenital lesions affecting approximately 5% of patients with NF1 but are the most common cause of long bone dysplasia and pseudoarthrosis.[85] Both children and adults with NF1 frequently have decreased bone mineral content compared with age-matched controls,[85,86] and osteoporosis occurs earlier than expected in postmenopausal women.[87]

Patients with scoliosis or tibial dysplasia/pseudoarthrosis should be referred to an orthopedist. Depending on the type and severity of scoliosis, bracing or surgical fusion may be required.[85] For limb dysplasia, total contact bracing can prevent fractures but, in the setting of fractures or pseudarthrosis, surgery is frequently needed.[85,88] Management of osteopenia and osteoporosis should focus on regular dual-energy X-ray absorptiometry (DEXA) scans as well as calcium and vitamin D supplementation.[89] The authors recommend DEXA screening starting at the age of 40 years and repeat scans based on the degree of bone loss.

Hypertension

Hypertension may develop in childhood and affects a large proportion of adults with NF1. Although primary (essential) hypertension is most common, NF1 increases the risk for secondary hypertension caused by moyamoya disease, renal artery stenosis, and pheochromocytoma.[90] Blood pressure should be monitored at least annually and, if clinically suspected, work-up initiated for secondary causes of hypertension including MRI and magnetic resonance angiogram of the abdomen.

Other malignancies

Patients with NF1 carry a higher risk of gastrointestinal stromal tumors, early-onset breast cancer, leukemia, and neuroendocrine tumors (eg, pheochromocytomas).[91] Notably, the increased breast cancer risk is specific to women <50 years old, in whom the standardized incidence ratio ranges from 4 to 11[92,93]; the risk in those ≥ 50 years old is similar to that in the general population.[92] Outcomes are poorer in NF1-associated breast cancer, presumably because of a higher incidence of triple-negative and human epidermal growth factor receptor 2 (HER2)-positive subtypes.[93] National Comprehensive Cancer Network (NCCN) guidelines recommend annual mammograms starting at age 30 years and to consider breast MRI between the ages of 30 and 50 years if there are any suspicious features. There is currently insufficient evidence to support the use of risk-reducing mastectomies in women with NF1, although this may be considered based on a positive family history or personal history of breast cancer.[92]

Prenatal and preimplantation genetic counseling

Patients with NF1 who wish to have children should receive preconception genetic counseling to discuss inheritance risks and the variability of the manifestations of the condition. Although many patients with NF1 proceed with natural conception, they should be informed of the range of reproductive options. For example, preimplantation genetic testing is a molecular technique whereby an embryo generated by in vitro fertilization is tested for a specific mutation before uterine transfer.[94] By contrast, prenatal testing is performed on fetal DNA during pregnancy. For both types of testing, knowledge of the affected parent's *NF1* mutation is required. Comprehensive genetic counseling should also include a discussion about alternative options.

SUMMARY

The neurofibromatoses are a group of related hereditary tumor predisposition syndromes that show phenotypic overlap with each other and other genetic syndromes. The presence of characteristic cutaneous features and certain types of tumors should raise suspicion for the possibility of NF1 and prompt clinicians to refer patients to the appropriate specialists familiar with NF1 and related conditions. This is necessary as manifestations of NF1 are highly variable, within and across patients, and there are important implications in determining optimal management for each individual with NF1 at each stage in their life.

REFERENCES

1. Evans DG, Howard E, Giblin C, et al. Birth incidence and prevalence of tumor-prone syndromes: estimates from a UK family genetic register service. Am J Med Genet A 2010;152A(2):327–32.
2. Kallionpaa RA, Uusitalo E, Leppavirta J, et al. Prevalence of neurofibromatosis type 1 in the Finnish population. Genet Med 2018;20(9):1082–6.
3. Uusitalo E, Leppavirta J, Koffert A, et al. Incidence and mortality of neurofibromatosis: a total population study in Finland. J Invest Dermatol 2015;135(3):904–6.
4. Rauen KA, Huson SM, Burkitt-Wright E, et al. Recent developments in neurofibromatoses and RASopathies: management, diagnosis and current and future therapeutic avenues. Am J Med Genet A 2015;167A(1):1–10.
5. Uusitalo E, Rantanen M, Kallionpaa RA, et al. Distinctive cancer associations in patients with neurofibromatosis type 1. J Clin Oncol 2016;34(17):1978–86.
6. Friedman JM. Epidemiology of neurofibromatosis type 1. Am J Med Genet 1999; 89(1):1–6.
7. Gutmann DH, Aylsworth A, Carey JC, et al. The diagnostic evaluation and multi-disciplinary management of neurofibromatosis 1 and neurofibromatosis 2. JAMA 1997;278(1):51–7.
8. National Institutes of Health consensus development conference statement: neurofibromatosis. Bethesda, Md., USA, July 13-15, 1987. Neurofibromatosis 1988;1(3):172–8.
9. Ferner RE, Gutmann DH. Neurofibromatosis type 1 (NF1): diagnosis and management. Handb Clin Neurol 2013;115:939–55.
10. DeBella K, Szudek J, Friedman JM. Use of the national institutes of health criteria for diagnosis of neurofibromatosis 1 in children. Pediatrics 2000;105(3 Pt 1): 608–14.
11. Wimmer K, Rosenbaum T, Messiaen L. Connections between constitutional mismatch repair deficiency syndrome and neurofibromatosis type 1. Clin Genet 2017;91(4):507–19.
12. Roberts AE, Allanson JE, Tartaglia M, et al. Noonan syndrome. Lancet 2013; 381(9863):333–42.
13. Evans DG, Moran A, King A, et al. Incidence of vestibular schwannoma and neurofibromatosis 2 in the North West of England over a 10-year period: higher incidence than previously thought. Otol Neurotol 2005;26(1):93–7.
14. Gareth Evans D, et al. Schwannomatosis: a genetic and epidemiologic study. J Neurol Neurosurg Psychiatry 2018.
15. Smith MJ, Bowers NL, Bulman M, et al. Revisiting neurofibromatosis type 2 diagnostic criteria to exclude LZTR1-related schwannomatosis. Neurology 2017; 88(1):87–92.
16. Evans DG. Neurofibromatosis type 2 (NF2): a clinical and molecular review. Orphanet J Rare Dis 2009;4:16.
17. Castellanos E, Plana A, Carrato C, et al. Early genetic diagnosis of neurofibromatosis type 2 from skin plaque plexiform schwannomas in childhood. JAMA Dermatol 2018;154(3):341–6.
18. McLaughlin ME, Pepin SM, Maccollin M, et al. Ocular pathologic findings of neurofibromatosis type 2. Arch Ophthalmol 2007;125(3):389–94.

19. Merker VL, Esparza S, Smith MJ, et al. Clinical features of schwannomatosis: a retrospective analysis of 87 patients. Oncologist 2012;17(10):1317–22.
20. MacCollin M, Chiocca EA, Evans DG, et al. Diagnostic criteria for schwannomatosis. Neurology 2005;64(11):1838–45.
21. Plotkin SR, Blakeley JO, Evans DG, et al. Update from the 2011 International Schwannomatosis Workshop: from genetics to diagnostic criteria. Am J Med Genet A 2013;161A(3):405–16.
22. Baser ME, Friedman JM, Evans DG. Increasing the specificity of diagnostic criteria for schwannomatosis. Neurology 2006;66(5):730–2.
23. Messiaen L, Yao S, Brems H, et al. Clinical and mutational spectrum of neurofibromatosis type 1-like syndrome. JAMA 2009;302(19):2111–8.
24. Pasmant E, Sabbagh A, Hanna N, et al. SPRED1 germline mutations caused a neurofibromatosis type 1 overlapping phenotype. J Med Genet 2009;46(7): 425–30.
25. Messiaen LM, Callens T, Mortier G, et al. Exhaustive mutation analysis of the NF1 gene allows identification of 95% of mutations and reveals a high frequency of unusual splicing defects. Hum Mutat 2000;15(6):541–55.
26. Skuse GR, Kosciolek BA, Rowley PT. Molecular genetic analysis of tumors in von Recklinghausen neurofibromatosis: loss of heterozygosity for chromosome 17. Genes Chromosomes Cancer 1989;1(1):36–41.
27. Weiss B, Bollag G, Shannon K. Hyperactive Ras as a therapeutic target in neurofibromatosis type 1. Am J Med Genet 1999;89(1):14–22.
28. Daston MM, Scrable H, Nordlund M, et al. The protein product of the neurofibromatosis type 1 gene is expressed at highest abundance in neurons, Schwann cells, and oligodendrocytes. Neuron 1992;8(3):415–28.
29. Ruggieri M, Huson SM. The clinical and diagnostic implications of mosaicism in the neurofibromatoses. Neurology 2001;56(11):1433–43.
30. Freret ME, Anastasaki C, Gutmann DH. Independent NF1 mutations underlie cafe-au-lait macule development in a woman with segmental NF1. Neurol Genet 2018;4(4):e261.
31. Shen MH, Harper PS, Upadhyaya M. Molecular genetics of neurofibromatosis type 1 (NF1). J Med Genet 1996;33(1):2–17.
32. Koczkowska M, Chen Y, Callens T, et al. Genotype-phenotype correlation in NF1: evidence for a more severe phenotype associated with missense mutations affecting NF1 codons 844-848. Am J Hum Genet 2018;102(1):69–87.
33. Kehrer-Sawatzki H, Mautner VF, Cooper DN. Emerging genotype-phenotype relationships in patients with large NF1 deletions. Hum Genet 2017;136(4):349–76.
34. Upadhyaya M, Huson SM, Davies M, et al. An absence of cutaneous neurofibromas associated with a 3-bp inframe deletion in exon 17 of the NF1 gene (c.2970-2972 delAAT): evidence of a clinically significant NF1 genotype-phenotype correlation. Am J Hum Genet 2007;80(1):140–51.
35. Quintans B, Pardo J, Campos B, et al. Neurofibromatosis without neurofibromas: confirmation of a genotype-phenotype correlation and implications for genetic testing. Case Rep Neurol 2011;3:86–90.
36. Koczkowska M, Callens T, Gomes A, et al. Expanding the clinical phenotype of individuals with a 3-bp in-frame deletion of the NF1 gene (c.2970_2972del): an update of genotype-phenotype correlation. Genet Med 2019;21(4):867–76.
37. Pinna V, Lanari V, Daniele P, et al. p.Arg1809Cys substitution in neurofibromin is associated with a distinctive NF1 phenotype without neurofibromas. Eur J Hum Genet 2015;23(8):1068–71.

38. Rojnueangnit K, Xie J, Gomes A, et al. High incidence of noonan syndrome features including short stature and pulmonic stenosis in patients carrying NF1 missense mutations affecting p.Arg1809: genotype-phenotype correlation. Hum Mutat 2015;36(11):1052–63.

39. Williams VC, Lucas J, Babcock MA, et al. Neurofibromatosis type 1 revisited. Pediatrics 2009;123(1):124–33.

40. Nunley KS, Gao F, Albers AC, et al. Predictive value of cafe au lait macules at initial consultation in the diagnosis of neurofibromatosis type 1. Arch Dermatol 2009;145(8):883–7.

41. Korf BR. Diagnostic outcome in children with multiple cafe au lait spots. Pediatrics 1992;90(6):924–7.

42. Fois A, Calistri L, Balestri P, et al. Relationship between cafe-au-lait spots as the only symptom and peripheral neurofibromatosis (NF1): a follow-up study. Eur J Pediatr 1993;152(6):500–4.

43. Hersh JH, American Academy of Pediatrics Committee on Genetics. Health supervision for children with neurofibromatosis. Pediatrics 2008;121(3):633–42.

44. Huson SM, Harper PS, Compston DA. Von Recklinghausen neurofibromatosis. A clinical and population study in south-east Wales. Brain 1988;111(Pt 6):1355–81.

45. Huson SM, Compston DA, Harper PS. A genetic study of von Recklinghausen neurofibromatosis in south east Wales. II. Guidelines for genetic counselling. J Med Genet 1989;26(11):712–21.

46. Ortonne N, Wolkenstein P, Blakeley JO, et al. Cutaneous neurofibromas: current clinical and pathologic issues. Neurology 2018;91(2 Supplement 1):S5–13.

47. Beert E, Brems H, Daniels B, et al. Atypical neurofibromas in neurofibromatosis type 1 are premalignant tumors. Genes Chromosomes Cancer 2011;50(12): 1021–32.

48. Roth TM, Petty EM, Barald KF. The role of steroid hormones in the NF1 phenotype: focus on pregnancy. Am J Med Genet A 2008;146A(12):1624–33.

49. Sbidian E, Duong TA, Valeyrie-Allanore L, et al. Neurofibromatosis type 1: neurofibromas and sex. Br J Dermatol 2016;174(2):402–4.

50. Brenaut E, Nizery-Guermeur C, Audebert-Bellanger S, et al. Clinical characteristics of pruritus in neurofibromatosis 1. Acta Derm Venereol 2016;96(3):398–9.

51. Wolkenstein P, Zeller J, Revuz J, et al. Quality-of-life impairment in neurofibromatosis type 1: a cross-sectional study of 128 cases. Arch Dermatol 2001;137(11): 1421–5.

52. Verma SK, Riccardi VM, Plotkin SR, et al. Considerations for development of therapies for cutaneous neurofibroma. Neurology 2018;91(2 Supplement 1):S21–30.

53. Cannon A, Chen MJ, Li P, et al. Cutaneous neurofibromas in Neurofibromatosis type I: a quantitative natural history study. Orphanet J Rare Dis 2018;13(1):31.

54. Lubs ML, Bauer MS, Formas ME, et al. Lisch nodules in neurofibromatosis type 1. N Engl J Med 1991;324(18):1264–6.

55. Parrozzani R, Pilotto E, Clementi M, et al. Retinal vascular abnormalities in a large cohort of patients affected by neurofibromatosis type 1: a study using optical coherence tomography angiography. Retina 2018;38(3):585–93.

56. Nguyen R, Dombi E, Widemann BC, et al. Growth dynamics of plexiform neurofibromas: a retrospective cohort study of 201 patients with neurofibromatosis 1. Orphanet J Rare Dis 2012;7:75.

57. Plotkin SR, Bredella MA, Cai W, et al. Quantitative assessment of whole-body tumor burden in adult patients with neurofibromatosis. PLoS One 2012;7(4): e35711.

58. Mautner VF, Hartmann M, Kluwe L, et al. MRI growth patterns of plexiform neuro-fibromas in patients with neurofibromatosis type 1. Neuroradiology 2006;48(3): 160–5.
59. Dombi E, Solomon J, Gillespie AJ, et al. NF1 plexiform neurofibroma growth rate by volumetric MRI: relationship to age and body weight. Neurology 2007;68(9): 643–7.
60. Mautner VF, Asuagbor FA, Dombi E, et al. Assessment of benign tumor burden by whole-body MRI in patients with neurofibromatosis 1. Neuro Oncol 2008;10(4): 593–8.
61. Stewart DR, Korf BR, Nathanson KL, et al. Care of adults with neurofibromatosis type 1: a clinical practice resource of the American College of Medical Genetics and Genomics (ACMG). Genet Med 2018;20(7):671–82.
62. Gross A, Wolters P, Baldwin A, et al. SPRINT: phase II study of the MEK 1/2 inhib-itor selumetinib (AZD244, ARRY-142886) in children with neurofibromatosis type 1 (NF1) and inoperable plexiform neurofibromas (PN): American Society for clinical oncology; 2018.
63. Farid M, Demicco EG, Garcia R, et al. Malignant peripheral nerve sheath tumors. Oncologist 2014;19(2):193–201.
64. Nguyen R, Jett K, Harris GJ, et al. Benign whole body tumor volume is a risk fac-tor for malignant peripheral nerve sheath tumors in neurofibromatosis type 1. J Neurooncol 2014;116(2):307–13.
65. Tucker T, Wolkenstein P, Revuz J, et al. Association between benign and malig-nant peripheral nerve sheath tumors in NF1. Neurology 2005;65(2):205–11.
66. King AA, Debaun MR, Riccardi VM, et al. Malignant peripheral nerve sheath tu-mors in neurofibromatosis 1. Am J Med Genet 2000;93(5):388–92.
67. De Raedt T, Brems H, Wolkenstein P, et al. Elevated risk for MPNST in NF1 micro-deletion patients. Am J Hum Genet 2003;72(5):1288–92.
68. Malbari F, Spira M, B Knight P, et al. Malignant peripheral nerve sheath tumors in neurofibromatosis: impact of family history. J Pediatr Hematol Oncol 2018;40(6): e359–63.
69. Reilly KM, Kim A, Blakely J, et al. Neurofibromatosis type 1-associated MPNST state of the science: outlining a research agenda for the future. J Natl Cancer Inst 2017;109(8). https://doi.org/10.1093/jnci/djx124.
70. Woodruff JM. Pathology of tumors of the peripheral nerve sheath in type 1 neuro-fibromatosis. Am J Med Genet 1999;89(1):23–30.
71. Wasa J, Nishida Y, Tsukushi S, et al. MRI features in the differentiation of malig-nant peripheral nerve sheath tumors and neurofibromas. AJR Am J Roentgenol 2010;194(6):1568–74.
72. Gupta G, Maniker A. Malignant peripheral nerve sheath tumors. Neurosurg Focus 2007;22(6):E12.
73. Higham CS, Dombi E, Rogiers A, et al. The characteristics of 76 atypical neuro-fibromas as precursors to neurofibromatosis 1 associated malignant peripheral nerve sheath tumors. Neuro Oncol 2018;20(6):818–25.
74. Ahlawat S, Fayad LM, Khan MS, et al. Current whole-body MRI applications in the neurofibromatoses: NF1, NF2, and schwannomatosis. Neurology 2016;87(7 Suppl 1):S31–9.
75. Ferner RE, Golding JF, Smith M, et al. [18F]2-fluoro-2-deoxy-D-glucose positron emission tomography (FDG PET) as a diagnostic tool for neurofibromatosis 1 (NF1) associated malignant peripheral nerve sheath tumours (MPNSTs): a long-term clinical study. Ann Oncology 2008;19(2):390–4.

76. Dunn GP, Spiliopoulos K, Plotkin SR, et al. Role of resection of malignant peripheral nerve sheath tumors in patients with neurofibromatosis type 1. J Neurosurg 2013;118(1):142–8.

77. Campen CJ, Gutmann DH. Optic pathway gliomas in neurofibromatosis type 1. J Child Neurol 2018;33(1):73–81.

78. Listernick R, Ferner RE, Liu GT, et al. Optic pathway gliomas in neurofibromatosis-1: controversies and recommendations. Ann Neurol 2007;61(3):189–98.

79. Ullrich NJ, Raja AI, Irons MB, et al. Brainstem lesions in neurofibromatosis type 1. Neurosurgery 2007;61(4):762–6 [discussion: 766–7].

80. Mahdi J, Shah AC, Sato A, et al. A multi-institutional study of brainstem gliomas in children with neurofibromatosis type 1. Neurology 2017;88(16):1584–9.

81. Rosenfeld A, Listernick R, Charrow J, et al. Neurofibromatosis type 1 and high-grade tumors of the central nervous system. Childs Nerv Syst 2010;26(5):663–7.

82. Strowd RE 3rd, Rodriguez FJ, McLendon RE, et al. Histologically benign, clinically aggressive: progressive non-optic pathway pilocytic astrocytomas in adults with NF1. Am J Med Genet A 2016;170(6):1455–61.

83. Hyman SL, Shores A, North KN. The nature and frequency of cognitive deficits in children with neurofibromatosis type 1. Neurology 2005;65(7):1037–44.

84. North KN, Riccardi V, Samango-Sprouse C, et al. Cognitive function and academic performance in neurofibromatosis. 1: consensus statement from the NF1 Cognitive Disorders Task Force. Neurology 1997;48(4):1121–7.

85. Delucia TA, Yohay K, Widmann RF. Orthopaedic aspects of neurofibromatosis: update. Curr Opin Pediatr 2011;23(1):46–52.

86. Brunetti-Pierri N, Doty SB, Hicks J, et al. Generalized metabolic bone disease in Neurofibromatosis type I. Mol Genet Metab 2008;94(1):105–11.

87. Kissil JL, Blakeley JO, Ferner RE, et al. What's new in neurofibromatosis? Proceedings from the 2009 NF Conference: new frontiers. Am J Med Genet A 2010;152A(2):269–83.

88. Stevenson DA, Little D, Armstrong L, et al. Approaches to treating NF1 tibial pseudarthrosis: consensus from the Children's Tumor Foundation NF1 Bone Abnormalities Consortium. J Pediatr Orthop 2013;33(3):269–75.

89. Elefteriou F, Kolanczyk M, Schindeler A, et al. Skeletal abnormalities in neurofibromatosis type 1: approaches to therapeutic options. Am J Med Genet A 2009; 149A(10):2327–38.

90. Kaas B, Huisman TA, Tekes A, et al. Spectrum and prevalence of vasculopathy in pediatric neurofibromatosis type 1. J Child Neurol 2013;28(5):561–9.

91. Walker L, Thompson D, Easton D, et al. A prospective study of neurofibromatosis type 1 cancer incidence in the UK. Br J Cancer 2006;95(2):233–8.

92. Daly MB, Pilarski R, Berry M, et al. NCCN guidelines insights: genetic/familial high-risk assessment: breast and ovarian, version 2.2017. J Natl Compr Canc Netw 2017;15(1):9–20.

93. Howell SJ, Hockenhull K, Salih Z, et al. Increased risk of breast cancer in neurofibromatosis type 1: current insights. Breast Cancer (Dove Med Press) 2017;9: 531–6.

94. Brezina PR, Brezina DS, Kearns WG. Preimplantation genetic testing. BMJ 2012; 345:e5908.

95. Miller DT, Freedenberg D, Schorry E, et al. AAP COUNCIL ON GENETICS, AAP AMERICAN COLLEGE OF MEDICAL GENETICS AND GENOMICS. Pediatrics 2019;143(5):e20190660.

Approach to Assessment of Parkinson Disease with Emphasis on Genetic Testing

Katelyn Payne, RN, CGC[a],*, Brooke Walls, MD[a],
Joanne Wojcieszek, MD[b]

KEYWORDS

• Parkinson disease • Genetics • Gene testing • *SNCA* • *LRRK* • *GBA*

KEY POINTS

- Parkinson disease (PD) is the second most common neurodegenerative disorder affecting 1% of persons more than 50 years of age and is caused by a combination of genetic and environmental factors.
- To date, there have been no therapies proved to slow the progression of PD. As genetic forms of PD are identified, there have been new targets for therapeutic intervention, and currently clinical trials for PARK-*LRRK2* and PARK-*GBA* are underway.
- With the emergence of clinical trials, it is important for health care providers to understand genetic testing for PD, when and how it should be ordered, and the benefit and risk to patients.
- Genetic test results may require further interpretation, and there are several available resources to guide clinicians, including the National Society of Genetic Counselors: Find a Genetic Counselor, Genetics Home Reference, OMIM, www.mdsgene.org, and GeneReviews.

Parkinson disease (PD) is a multifactorial syndrome with age-associated penetrance for which genetic susceptibility and environmental exposure contribute to risk. It is the second most common neurodegenerative disorder, following Alzheimer disease, affecting 1% of persons more than 50 years of age. Incidence in persons more than 40 years of age is 37 per 100,000 in women and 61 per 100,000 in men.[1]

It is estimated that there are more than 1 million persons with PD the United States. The average age of onset is approximately 60 years. PD is divided into 2 categories: late-onset PD, presenting after age 50 years, and early-onset PD, presenting before

Disclosure: Clinical trial support by Vaccinex.
[a] Department of Neurology, Indiana University School of Medicine, 355 West 16th Street, Suite 4700, Indianapolis, IN 46202, USA; [b] Indiana University School of Medicine, 355 West 16th Street, Suite 4700, Indianapolis, IN 46202, USA
* Corresponding author.
E-mail address: paynekk@iu.edu

Med Clin N Am 103 (2019) 1055–1075
https://doi.org/10.1016/j.mcna.2019.08.003
0025-7125/19/© 2019 Elsevier Inc. All rights reserved.

age 50 years. Within the early-onset group, there is the extremely rare young-onset PD with symptoms before age 20 years.

Primary care providers are called on to diagnose and treat the early to middle-stage symptoms of PD. Patients are referred to movement disorder specialists often to confirm the diagnosis and later in the disease when symptoms become more complex. The disorder begins insidiously with unilateral resting tremor, stiffness (rigidity), and slowness (bradykinesia). As the disease progresses, patients develop bilateral symptoms, balance disturbances, and other complications such as levodopa-induced dyskinesia (50%), motor fluctuations (50%), dementia (30%), and hallucinations (50%). There should be robust and persistent response to levodopa for at least 5 years. The survival rate in PD at 10 years is similar to that of the general population, whereas after 10 years there is a modest increase in mortality. Factors that are associated with higher mortality include male gender, absence of tremor at disease onset, and gait impairment.[2]

To date, there have been no therapies proved to slow the progression of PD. Neuroprotective trials have invariably failed because of poor understanding of the underlying pathogenesis. It is not surprising that a single therapy may not influence progression given the heterogeneous nature of this condition. PD is caused by loss of dopamine-producing neurons in the substantia nigra. The recent identification of genetic subtypes of PD has led to better understanding of the diverse underlying cellular defects leading to neuronal death, including various proportions of mitochondrial dysfunction, impaired processing of proteins within lysosomes and proteasomes, oxidative stress, inflammation, and environmental insult.[3]

There is increasing availability of genetic testing for PD but there are few recommendations on how these tests should be used in clinical practice. This article guides clinicians on the overall management of patients with PD, with emphasis on determining which patients should have genetic testing and how to interpret those results.

CLINICAL ASPECTS

PD is diagnosed clinically based on the presence of bradykinesia with either resting tremor or rigidity.[4]

Patients report a tremor that is present when the limb is not engaged in movement (resting tremor), such as when watching TV, and typically disappears with action. Some patients note onset of tremor with posture; for example, when holding a phone. Patients may report small handwriting (micrographia) or reduced fine motor dexterity (eg, typing). Speech may become soft (hypophonia).

Family members may notice reduced facial expression (masked facies) or reduced blinking (hypomimia). PD does not cause slurred speech (dysarthria). There may be slowness of overall body movement, such as difficulty getting in and out of a car or trouble rolling over in bed.

The examination of a patient with suspected PD should include observing the patient sitting on the examination table with legs dangling so as to see a resting tremor of the foot (may not be present when the foot is planted against the floor). The hands should be in a relaxed posture placed on either thigh. Sometimes, a chin tremor or even unilateral facial tremor can be seen in this relaxed pose. Tone of the neck and limbs should be tested by passively moving the wrist, elbow, and knee looking for cogwheel rigidity. Limb bradykinesia can be tested by performing finger tapping, opening and closing of the hands, or foot tapping. The clinician is looking for slowness of tapping but also irregularity or fatigability. Ask the patients to write their names repeatedly to see whether micrographia occurs with prolonged exertion. Ask the patients to fold their arms in front of the body and stand without pushing up from the chair. The patient should walk down the hall and the examiner looks for reduced arm swing or dragging of a leg. True resting tremor often appears when the patient is walking and the arm is totally relaxed. In addition, check for postural reflexes to see whether the patient can recover from a pull backward. PD is staged per the Hoehn and Yahr scale (**Box 1**).

The remainder of the neurologic examination should be normal. The presence of other signs suggests an alternative diagnosis (**Table 1**).

The range of extraocular movement should be full; limitations raise the possibility of progressive supranuclear palsy (PSP) or stroke. Muscle power should be full. There should be no Babinski sign, and if present this suggests multiple system atrophy (MSA), Parkinson type (MSA-P), corticobasal syndrome (CBS), or stroke. Many patients with MSA-P can resemble PD early in their course but also have prominent early autonomic symptoms, such as syncope, urinary incontinence, and violaceous discoloration of the hands and feet. Significant cognitive dysfunction at the time of motor symptom onset suggests dementia with Lewy bodies (DLB).

Wilson disease (WD) should always be excluded in persons less than 50 years old with new parkinsonism because it is a potentially treatable disease that is otherwise lethal if undiagnosed. WD is a disorder of impaired copper excretion in which the liver is not able to dispose of excess copper in the bile. WD can be diagnosed in several ways, 2 of which are (1) increased copper excretion, as measured by 24-hour urinary copper collection (performed only through a highly reputable laboratory in a copper-free container), and (2) Kayser-Fleischer rings found on slit lamp examination plus low serum ceruloplasmin level. For more information on WD, see the accompanying article on the genetics of liver disease in this issue.

Neuroimaging

The diagnostic evaluation of PD typically includes brain MRI, which is normal early in disease but can provide evidence of an alternative diagnosis such as normal-pressure hydrocephalus or infarction. If there are no atypical features, imaging can be waived.

Although the diagnosis of PD remains clinical, there are instances of diagnostic uncertainty, especially in early stages of disease, and neuroimaging such as dopamine transporter (DAT) with single-photon emission computed tomography (SPECT) or ^{18}F-DOPA (L-6-[^{18}F]fluoro-3,4-dihydroxyphenylalanine) can be used to make a more definitive diagnosis of dopaminergic deficit.

DAT-SPECT was approved by the US Food and Drug Administration in 2011 and is readily available as a clinical nuclear medicine test. This imaging technique uses a

---

Box 1
Hoehn and Yahr staging

1. Unilateral involvement with minimal or no functional disability

2. Bilateral or midline involvement with normal postural reflexes

3. Mild to moderate disability, impaired postural reflexes, but still functionally independent

4. Severe disability, but able to walk and stand without assistance

5. Bedbound or wheelchair bound unless assisted

Adapted from Hoehn MM, Yahr MD. Parkinsonism: onset, progression and mortality. Neurology 1967;17(5):427–42.

Table 1
Differential diagnosis of parkinsonism

Diagnosis	Comments
Wilson Disease	Must be ruled out in all patients <50 y old (see text)
Drug-induced parkinsonism	Dopamine receptor blocking agents (antipsychotics, antiemetics) reserpine, tetrabenazine, lithium, flunarizine, cinnarizine
Depression with psychomotor slowing/catatonia	Bradykinesia, waxy flexibility; no tremor
Dementia with Lewy bodies	Early hallucinations, fluctuations in mentation
Progressive supranuclear palsy	Early falls, dysarthria, dysphagia, apathy, impaired vertical eye movements (downgaze)
Multiple system atrophy, Parkinson type	Early autonomic instability
Corticobasal syndrome	Apraxia, myoclonus, sensory loss, alien limb
Vascular parkinsonism	Lower body parkinsonism, hyperreflexia
Huntington disease	Chorea, motor impersistence, slow saccades
Toxins	Carbon monoxide, manganese, mercury, cyanide, methanol, organophosphates, MPTP
Viral encephalitis	HIV, Coxsackie, Japanese B, St Louis, West Nile
Paraneoplastic encephalitis	Abrupt onset, behavioral changes, seizures
Prion disease, such as Creutzfeldt-Jakob disease	Rapid-onset dementia, myoclonic jerks, ataxia
Dystonic limb tremor	Dystonia is the primary finding
Psychogenic/conversion disorder	Abrupt onset, intermittent, variable appearance, abates with distraction

Abbreviations: HIV, human immunodeficiency virus; MPTP, 1-methyl-4-phenyl-1,2,3,6-tetrahydropyridine.

dopamine-related ligand in combination with SPECT to evaluate the function of the DAT protein found on presynaptic dopaminergic neurons. In PD, there is a loss of dopaminergic neurons within the striatum and there are reduced levels of the DAT protein in these areas.[5] Sensitivity and specificity of DAT-SPECT are 78% and 97%, respectively.[6]

^{18}F-DOPA is an agent used with PET to measure the amount of presynaptic dopaminergic neurons.[7] ^{18}F-DOPA serves as a dopamine precursor and is taken up by the presynaptic dopaminergic neuron. Thus, it serves as a marker for the loss of dopaminergic neurons. ^{18}F-DOPA PET has a sensitivity of 95.4% and specificity of 100% but has limited availability because of the need for a cyclotron to generate this isotope.[8]

Both of these imaging modalities show a rostrocaudal pattern of dopaminergic cell loss, starting in the putamen on the contralateral side of symptom onset, and progressing to the ipsilateral caudate and eventually becoming bilateral.[9] DAT-SPECT and ^{18}F-DOPA are helpful in distinguishing parkinsonism from essential tremor, dystonic tremor, psychogenic (nonphysiologic) tremor, drug-induced parkinsonism, vascular parkinsonism, and dopa-responsive dystonia. However, they cannot distinguish PD from MSA, PSP, or CBS.[9–11]

Symptomatic Treatment

Once the diagnosis of PD has been made, the next step is to determine whether the patient's symptoms are sufficiently bothersome to initiate treatment. Levodopa continues to be the most effective medication available but long-term use can cause dyskinesias and hallucinations. Dopamine agonists (pramipexole, ropinirole, rotigotine) can also be first line for motor symptoms; however, patients should be monitored for development of impulse control disorder and excessive daytime sleepiness. Anticholinergics (trihexyphenidyl, benztropine) are effective but often underused. They should be avoided in elderly patients because of their potential for causing hallucinations, worsening constipation, and confusion. Amantadine can be used to help tremor and dyskinesia. Monoamine oxidase B inhibitors (selegiline, rasagiline, safinamide) may provide modest benefit in treating the motor symptoms of PD. Catechol-O-methyltransferase inhibitors (entacapone) may be used as an adjunct to extend the duration of each levodopa dose. When PD symptoms begin to interfere with daily activities, work, or hobbies, then deep brain stimulation (DBS) or continuous intestinal levodopa infusion can be considered.

INTRODUCTION TO GENETICS OF PARKINSON DISEASE

The cause of PD eluded science until 1990 when Golbe and colleagues[12] described 2 Italian families (the Contoursi kindred) with autosomal dominant (AD) PD. Before this, PD was considered a sporadic disorder, even though approximately 10% to 15% of patients reported a positive family history. In 1997, the gene causing PD in these families was identified (SNCA), and it encoded a previously unstudied protein called alpha-synuclein.[13] The initial SNCA gene abnormality was a single point mutation. It was later discovered that patients could develop PD from having an excessive amount of normal or wild-type alpha-synuclein protein caused by triplication of the gene.[14] This groundbreaking discovery was the first evidence that a single gene without environmental trigger could cause PD. It was soon discovered that alpha-synuclein was a major component of the Lewy body.

Although alpha-synuclein mutations are rare and represent a small proportion of heritable PD, identification of this novel protein and study of its role in cellular function has formidably increased the understanding PD. Mutations in alpha-synuclein alter the structure of the protein making it prone to misfolding and aggregation. Abnormal folding, excessive amounts, or inadequate clearance of alpha-synuclein play a role in neuronal death. In sporadic PD, alpha-synuclein is likely a major participant in the pathogenesis of the disorder, possibly through reduced clearance. Targeted therapeutic interventions using active and passive immunity to reduce the amount of alpha-synuclein accumulation are under investigation[15] (ClinicalTrials.gov: NCT02267434).

Another major development in the genetics of PD came in 2003 when it was observed that some patients with Gaucher disease (GD) had parkinsonism,[16] followed by the astounding discovery that mutations in the GBA gene were a major risk factor for PD.[17] GD is an autosomal recessive (AR) lysosomal storage disorder caused by mutations in the GBA gene, which encodes the glucocerebrosidase enzyme and is responsible for breaking down glucocerebroside into glucose and ceramide. GBA mutations greatly reduce glucocerebrosidase activity, leading to an accumulation of byproducts that become toxic to normal cell function and represent significant risk for PD. GBA mutations are classified as mild (eg, N370S) or severe (eg, L444P) based on the amount of residual enzyme activity. Individuals with GD have a 5% to 7% chance of developing PD before age 70 years and a 9% to 12% chance by age 80 years.[18]

Discovering the link between GD and PD turned the spotlight on the role of lysosomes in the pathogenesis of PD and has provided new targets for therapeutic intervention. Clinical trials for patients with PD who carry a *GBA* mutation are now underway (www.clinicaltrials.gov: NCT02906020), which introduces a potential motivation for patients to learn whether they carry a *GBA* mutation. Testing for the common N370S mutation is available via direct-to-consumer (DTC) testing or more formally through a health care provider.

Clinical Aspects of Parkinson Disease Susceptibility Genes

Most cases of PD are sporadic with no family history of the disorder. The risk to develop PD increases with age, affecting 1% of the population more than age 55 years, 3% more than age 75 years, and 5% more than age 85 years. In sporadic cases, the risk to first-degree relatives to develop PD is 3% to 7% over their lifetimes. The most influential risk factor for PD is having a positive family history.[19,20]

Inherited PD (meaning PD caused by mutation in a single gene) accounts for 5% to 10% of all cases with AD, AR, and X-linked inheritance reported.[21,22] To date, there are at least 19 genes associated with an increased risk of developing PD.[21] The following genes can cause parkinsonism that resembles late-onset, sporadic PD: *SNCA*, *LRRK2*, *GBA*, *PRKN*, *DJ-1*, and *PINK1*.

Previously, there was a distinction between mendelian (monogenic) forms of PD and susceptibility loci (eg, *GBA*). The distinction has blurred because incomplete penetrance has been identified in most PD genes, and, within each gene, specific mutations have different degrees of penetrance.[23] For these reasons, this article refers to all gene mutations associated with PD as genetic risk factors.

Historically, PARK designations were used to label types of PD when a chromosome region had been discovered but an exact gene had not been identified.[24,25] In 2016, the International Parkinson and Movement Disorder Society Task Force for Nomenclature of Genetic Movement Disorders recommended standardized nomenclature for the naming of genetically determined parkinsonism in which the phenotype prefix, PARK, is followed by the italicized official gene symbol (eg, PARK-*LRRK2*).[24]

The list of genes in **Table 2** includes genetic risk factors of PD for which there is testing clinically available and in which parkinsonism is the primary manifestation. *PARK* loci are listed when available.

Autosomal Dominant Genes

AD forms of PD are more likely to be associated with incomplete penetrance and variable age of onset. In general, as the frequency of monogenic variants increases in the population, the penetrance decreases; the rarer the variant, the higher the disease penetrance.[25]

The currently known genes associated with AD PD include PARK-*SNCA*, PARK-*LRRK2*, *GBA*, PARK-*UCH-L1*, PARK-*VPS35*, PARK-*EIF4G1*, PARK-*HTRA2*, PARK-*CHCHD2*, and PARK-*DNAJ13*.

PARK-SNCA

SNCA mutations are a rare cause of PD occurring in less than 1% of cases, mostly in families from Italy, Greece, Spain, and Germany. As mentioned earlier, the *SNCA* gene encodes the alpha-synuclein protein, which likely plays a role in maintaining presynaptic terminals and regulating dopamine release. Two different types of *SNCA* gene alterations have been identified in PD: point mutations (PARK1) and duplications or triplications of the gene (PARK4). Both types of alterations cause aggregation of an abnormal protein product that forms Lewy bodies. The protein aggregates become toxic to neurons through multiple mechanisms, including endoplasmic reticulum overload and mitochondrial cell death. Alpha-synuclein is likely a major participant in the

Table 2
Parkinson disease genetic risk factors

Mode of Inheritance	Gene Name	PD Locus	Early Onset (<50 y)	Late Onset (>50 y)
AD	SNCA	PARK1 (mutations) PARK4 (duplications and triplications)	X	X
	LRRK2	PARK8	—	X
	GBA	No PARK locus	X	X
	UCHL1	PARK5	X	X
	VPS35	PARK17	—	X
	EIF4G1	PARK18	—	X
	HTRA2	PARK13	X	X
	CHCHD2	PARK22	X	X
	DNAJC13	No PARK locus	—	X
AR	PRKN	PARK2	X	—
	PINK1	PARK6	X	—
	DJ-1	PARK7	X	—
	ATP13A2	PARK9	X	—
	FBX07	PARK15	X	—
	SLC6A3	SLC6A3	X	—
	PLA2G6	PARK14	X	X
	DNAJC6	PARK19	X	—
	SYNJ1	PARK20	X	—
	VPS13 C	PARK23	X	—
X linked	TAF1	PARK12	—	X

pathogenesis of both sporadic and monogenic forms of PD. SNCA mutations can mimic DLB and MSA.[26]

Disease phenotype (ie, clinical characteristics) and penetrance of PARK-SNCA are specific to the type of SNCA mutation. In the Contoursi kindred, affected individuals had an SNCA point mutation (G209A),[13] an average age of diagnosis of 46.5 years, and a rapid course that averaged 9.7 years from symptom onset to death. The clinical presentation and response to levodopa were typical for late-onset PD. More recent analysis of 5 specific point mutations (A30P, E46K, H50Q, G51D, and A53T) suggests a later disease onset of 49 years.[23]

SNCA gene duplications have a median age of onset of 48 years and a low disease penetrance of 33%.[23] SNCA gene triplications have a median age of onset of 39 years and a more aggressive disease course. Clinical features include a resting tremor, dysautonomia, levodopa responsiveness, cognitive dysfunction, and rapid disease progression. SNCA gene triplications can present as DLB with death occurring 2 to 12 years after symptom onset.[23,25] This rare form of PD would not be detected by traditional nucleotide sequencing, but a gene panel that includes deletion/duplication analysis would detect an extra copy of the SNCA gene.

PARK-LRRK2

LRRK2 is the most common genetic cause of PD, being associated with both genetic and sporadic forms.[27] The LRRK2 gene was first identified in Basque families with AD PD in 2004 and encodes a protein known as dardarin, or leucine-rich repeat kinase 2.[28,29] LRRK2 functions as a kinase assisting in phosphorylation, thereby playing an important role in turning on and turning off cell pathways. It is also involved in regulating autophagy, a cellular process that presents cell constituents to the lysosome for degradation. Disease-causing *LRRK2* mutations lead to excessive kinase activity and impaired lysosomal function.[30]

The clinical manifestations of PARK-*LRRK2* are typically indistinguishable from late-onset sporadic PD. The motor symptoms (eg, disease severity, rate of progression, dyskinesia) and nonmotor symptoms (eg, cognition, olfaction) of PARK-*LRRK2* are more benign than those of sporadic PD. Less common features include early age of onset, dystonia, amyotrophy, DLB, and frontotemporal dementia. Disease duration is shorter for patients with PARK-*LRRK2* compared with sporadic (11 years vs 15 years).[31]

Although many *LRRK2* mutations have been documented, only 6 (G2019S, R1441C, R1441G, R1441H, I2020T, and Y1699C) are unequivocally linked to disease[25] and 2 others (R1628P and G2385R) are clinically relevant sequence variants. Some specific characteristics of each of these have been identified:

G2019S

One specific *LRRK2* founder mutation, G2019S, is identified in 5% to 7% of familial PD cases and 1% to 2% of sporadic cases.[31,32] This founder mutation is most prevalent in individuals of Ashkenazi Jewish and North African Berber Arab ancestry. G2019S accounts for 15% to 20% of PD in Ashkenazi Jewish individuals, 30% to 40% of PD in North African Berber Arabs, and 1% of PD in northern European white people.[33,34] Penetrance is variable and influenced by age, gender, and ethnic background.

In 2008, the risk of developing PD with the G2019S mutation was reported as 28% at age 59 years, 51% at age 69 years, and 74% at age 79 years.[31] In the North African Berber Arab population, the penetrance of the G2019S mutation is 20% by age 50 years, but greater than 80% by age 70 years.[33,35] More recently, penetrance by age 80 years in non-Ashkenazi Jewish individuals was estimated at 42.5% compared with 25% in Ashkenazi Jewish individuals.[36]

R1441G/A1441C

Position 1441 in the *LRRK2* gene is the second most common site for mutations. The R1441G mutation is responsible for 46% of familial PD and for 2.5% of sporadic PD in people of Basque descent. Lifetime penetrance of the R1441G mutation is 13% at age 65 years and increases to 83% at age 80 years with no difference in gender.[37] The A1441C mutation is most frequent in individuals of Belgian ancestry.

R1628P and G2385R

These mutations are considered common risk factors for PD in Asians. Each mutation doubles the risk of PD and was present in 4% of controls, 7% of patients with late-onset PD, 10% with early-onset PD, and 23% with familial PD in this Chinese cohort from Taiwan.[38] Farrer and colleagues[38] suggested that the G2385R variant may be the most common risk factor for both early-onset and late-onset PD worldwide when considering the size of the Asian population.

Reducing *LRRK2* kinase activity has become the target of a specific *LRRK2* disease-modifying therapy (http://denalitherapeutics.com/press). Such trials not only may benefit patients with *LRRK2*-related PD but also may be applied to sporadic PD. Potential participation in such targeted clinical trials may serve as an impetus for some patients with sporadic PD to learn their gene status. There is DTC testing available for the G2019S mutation, or patients can have more extensive genetic testing, including full gene sequencing, through their medical practitioners.

GBA

Approximately 7% to 15% of individuals with PD carry a *GBA* mutation, with higher rates in the Ashkenazi Jewish population. Depending on the *GBA* mutation, penetrance is generally less than that of *LRRK2* mutations. For carriers of a single *GBA* mutation, penetrance estimates vary from 6% in individuals with a mild mutation to up to 24% in individuals with a severe mutation. Patients with PD with a *GBA* mutation are more likely to have earlier age of onset of parkinsonism (age 53 years for severe *GBA* mutation and age 58 years for mild mutations). Most reports suggest more severe motor symptoms but there seems to be good levodopa responsiveness. *GBA* mutation carriers with PD have earlier onset and higher incidence of dementia compared with sporadic PD, and the clinical picture can resemble DLB (may be mutation dependent).[39–43]

PARK-UCH-L1

The *UCH-L1* gene encodes the ubiquitin–C-terminal hydrolase L1 and is a rare cause of PD. This gene was first described in 2 German siblings with symptom onset at ages 49 and 51 years and progression similar to sporadic PD.[44] A paternal uncle and paternal grandmother were also affected, but their father was unaffected, suggesting incomplete penetrance.

UCH-L1, along with PRKN, are critical for protein processing in the cell through their role in the ubiquitin proteasome system (UPS). The function of the UPS is to degrade unwanted or abnormal proteins (termed ubiquitination). This process serves as a signal to move unneeded proteins into specialized structures known as proteasomes, where the proteins are degraded by proteolysis. Failure of this disposal system can lead to buildup of excess, damaged, or misshapen proteins that disrupt normal cellular homeostasis and can lead to cell death. *UCH-L1* is necessary for the maintenance of axonal health and stability, and its loss results in axonal degeneration and neuronal death.

PARK-VPS35

The *VPS35* gene encodes for a Golgi trafficking protein. The D620N mutation was described in Swiss and Austrian families with average age of onset of 51 years and clinical presentation similar to sporadic PD with tremor predominance and good response to levodopa. In these families, there was age-dependent, incomplete penetrance of PD.[45,46] This gene is found primarily in white people and is rare in Asians, except in Japanese.

PARK-EIF4G1

The *EIF4G1* gene encodes for the eukaryotic translation initiation factor 4-gamma 1 protein involved in messenger RNA translation during periods of cell stress. This condition resembles levodopa-responsive sporadic PD with a mild course and no significant cognitive impairment.[47]

PARK-HTRA2

The *HTRA2* gene encodes a serine protease within mitochondria that mediates cell death and was described in 4 German patients with typical PD, and mean age of onset was 57 years.[48,49]

PARK-CHCHD2

The *CHCHD2* gene encodes a transcription factor that is involved in the electron transport chain.[50] Patients had a mean onset at 55 years with typical levodopa-responsive PD.[51]

PARK-DNAJC13

This gene encodes an endosomal protein involved in vesicular trafficking. Mean age of onset is 67 years and patients are levodopa responsive with a slowly progressive course.[52]

Autosomal Recessive Genes

AR forms of PD are more common in offspring of consanguineous relationships. The phenotype involves an earlier age of onset, slow disease progression, and mild non-motor symptoms. Atypical and juvenile forms of PD are typically recessively inherited.[25] There is increasing evidence that carriers of 1 AR mutation may have a slightly increased risk for PD later in life.[53] The currently known genes associated with AR PD include *PRKN* (PARK2), *PINK-1* (PARK6), *DJ-1* (PARK7), *ATP13A2* (PARK9), *FBXO7* (PARK15), SLC6A3, *PLA2G6* (PARK14), *DNAJC6* (PARK19), *SYNJ1* (PARK20), and *VPS13C* (PARK23).

PARK-PRKN

The *PRKN* gene encodes for the cytoplasmic protein, parkin, an E3 ubiquitin ligase that helps eliminate dysfunctional mitochondria and unwanted proteins within the cell. Parkin dysfunction leads to accumulation of excess protein and mitochondria, ultimately resulting in cell death. A unique feature of this PD subtype is that it is generally not associated with the presence of Lewy bodies.[54] The *PRKN* mutation represents the most common AR cause of PD, with a prevalence of 49% in young-onset PD, and a 77% prevalence in patients younger than 20 years. The phenotype is characterized by early dystonia, symmetric parkinsonism at onset, and hyperreflexia; dementia is rare. These patients respond well to levodopa but usually have dyskinesia and early motor fluctuations.[55] Although PARK-*PRKN* is considered an AR disorder, heterozygous mutations may be a risk factor for PD.[56]

PARK-PINK1

The *PINK-1* gene encodes the PTEN-induced putative kinase 1 protein. During periods of cell stress, the PINK-1 protein phosphorylates mitochondrial proteins, labeling them for ubiquitination by parkin for elimination from the cell.[3,57,58] This parkinsonism is slowly progressive, asymmetrical, responds well to levodopa,[59] and accounts for 3.7% of cases of early-onset PD.[3]

PARK-DJ-1

The *DJ-1* gene encodes a transcription regulation protein that protects against oxidative stress, especially in the mitochondria. Protein malfunction results in death of dopaminergic neurons.[60,61] PARK-*DJ-1* is rare and is characterized by spasticity, hyperreflexia, dystonia, supranuclear gaze palsy, and good levodopa response.[3]

PARK-ATP13A2

The *ATP13A2* gene encodes for the 5 P-type ATPase protein that plays a role in lysosomal function. Mutations of this protein result in reduced clearance of abnormal mitochondria and accumulation of alpha-synuclein within the cell.[3,62] PARK-*ATP13A2* is a very rare form of juvenile-onset PD. Patients have spasticity, hyperreflexia, supranuclear gaze palsy, and dementia. There is an initial response to levodopa but then early development of dyskinesias and hallucinations.[62]

PARK-FBXO7

The *FBXO7* gene encodes for the Skp1-Cullin-F-Box type E3 ligase (FBXO7) protein, which plays a role in regulation of mitochondrial function during oxidative stress.[63] FBXO7 dysfunction prevents elimination of abnormal mitochondria, resulting in cell death.[64] This juvenile-onset PD presents with hyperreflexia and spasticity. There is a variable response to levodopa and a long disease course.[65]

PARK-SLC6A3

Mutations in the *SLC6A3* gene result in loss of function of the DAT found on presynaptic dopaminergic neurons, leading to impaired reuptake of dopamine. It is associated with infantile parkinsonism-dystonia.[66] These patients present in infancy with parkinsonism or hyperkinetic movements, dystonia, abnormal eye movements, and pyramidal symptoms, but are cognitively intact. They are often misdiagnosed with cerebral palsy. They do not respond well to levodopa, but may have some early benefit from dopamine agonists. One patient even underwent DBS therapy with some benefit.[67] This form of parkinsonism is very rare, with only 30 reported cases as of 2017.[68]

PARK-PLA2G6

PLA2G6 encodes for the protein calcium-independent phospholipase A2, group VI, which is involved in oxidative stress response and elimination of dysfunctional mitochondria.[3] This gene has been associated with infantile neuroaxonal dystrophy, neurodegeneration with brain iron accumulation type 2, and adult-onset levodopa-responsive dystonia-parkinsonism.[69]

PARK-DNAJC6

DNAJC6 encodes for auxilin, which plays a role in synaptic vesicle recycling.[70] This very rare juvenile-onset PD includes poor response to levodopa and rapid disease progression, causing patients to become wheelchair bound within a few years. There is also hyperreflexia, spasticity, seizures, cognitive impairment, and dystonia.[71,72] Another phenotypic variant of *DNAJC6* can cause onset of levodopa-responsive parkinsonism in the third to fourth decades and is more slowly progressive.[73]

PARK-SYNJ1

The *SYNJ1* gene codes for synaptojanin-1 (SYNJ1), a phosphoinositide phosphatase that, along with auxilin, plays a role in synaptic vesicle recycling. Krebs and colleagues[74] and Quadri and colleagues[75] both discovered this abnormal gene function in 2013 in 2 Iranian siblings and 2 Italian siblings, respectively. These patients were found to have early-onset PD with initial response to levodopa but then developed early dyskinesia. The Iranian patients had seizures, whereas the Italian siblings had cognitive dysfunction.

PARK-VPS13C

This mutation was found in 3 unrelated patients who developed parkinsonism between the ages of 25 and 46 years. There is initial short-lived response to levodopa, followed by rapid progression to a bedridden state with dementia, dysautonomia, and pyramidal signs.[76]

X-linked Genes

PARK-TAF1

Only 1 form of X-linked PD has been identified to date. It is rare and associated with the *TAF1* gene; men tend to be more severely affected than women. *TAF1* mutations are associated with dystonia-parkinsonism. Parkinsonism typically appears first, and dystonia becomes evident later in the disease course. One particular mutation in the *TAF1* gene has been identified in individuals of Filipino ancestry.[77]

Overlapping genetic disorders

Parkinsonism can be a primary or secondary feature in a variety of genetic disorders described here.

Dopa-responsive dystonias

Dopa-responsive dystonias are caused by deficiencies of proteins involved in the dopamine synthesis pathway, including (GTP-cyclohydrolase-1, tyrosine hydroxylase, sepiapterin reductase, and 6-pyruvoyl tetrahydropterin). GTP-cyclohydrolase-1 deficiency can be either AD (DYT5a: Segawa disease) or AR, whereas the others are recessive. These dystonias present from infancy to adulthood with primary dystonia that is robustly levodopa responsive. There may be parkinsonism with postural instability. Symptoms classically improve with sleep (diurnal variation).[78]

Fragile X tremor/ataxia syndrome

Fragile X tremor/ataxia syndrome (FXTAS) occurs in patients who are carriers of the *FMR1* premutation allele on the X chromosome. A premutation is characterized by 50 to 200 CGG repeats within this gene, and a full expansion greater than 200 repeats causes fragile X syndrome.[79] Prevalence of carriers for the premutation has been reported as 1 in 259 women and 1 in 813 men.[80,81] Typically, affected men present in their 50s with mixed-type tremor and cerebellar ataxia.[82] There is variability in presentation and some patients present with tremor and bradykinesia resembling PD,[83,84] or with autonomic dysfunction, gait imbalance, or ophthalmoplegia that may resemble MSA or PSP.[85,86] There can be cognitive impairment, sleep dysfunction, and peripheral neuropathy.[83] Brain MRI may show T2 hyperintensities of the corpus callosum (splenium) and middle cerebellar peduncles, both of which should prompt consideration for FXTAS.[87]

Spinocerebellar ataxias

Of the 30 types of spinocerebellar ataxia (SCA), those that include parkinsonism are SCAs 2, 3, 6, 8, 12, 17, and 21, all of which are AD. SCAs 2 and 3 may be levodopa responsive.[88] **Table 3** lists the distinguishing characteristics among the SCAs with parkinsonism.

Genetic testing strategy

Historically, the approach to genetic testing involved sending individual gene tests in a serial fashion based on highest probability. More recently, it has become more cost-effective and efficient to send panels that include not only PD genes but also related disorders. Clinically available testing includes panels with (1) full gene sequencing that detects DNA substitutions, insertions, and small deletions, and (2) copy number analysis that detects larger duplications and deletions, as can be seen in PARK-*SNCA* and PARK-*PRKN*. It is important to understand that not all changes identified are clinically relevant, and, if a mutation or variant of uncertain significance is identified, it may require further results interpretation.

Table 3
Spinocerebellar ataxias associated with parkinsonism

Type	Mean Age of Onset (y)	Distinguishing Features	Mutation
SCA 2	35	Hypoactive reflexes, facial myokymia, dystonia[89]	CAG expansion within ATXN2
SCA 3 type IV associated with parkinsonism	37	"Bulging eyes" hyperactive reflexes, peripheral neuropathy[90,91]	CAG expansion with ATXN3
SCA 6	43–52	Slowly progressive, intention tremor, dystonia, blepharospasm[92,93]	CAG expansion within CACNA1A gene
SCA 8	—	Slowly progressive, ataxia and imbalance at onset, may have cognitive changes, may have seizures[94]	CTG expansion within ATXN8OS, and CAG expansion within ATXN8
SCA 12	40	Upper extremity tremor, head tremor (often initially diagnosed at essential tremor), cognitive changes, only mild cerebellar dysfunction[95,96]	CAG repeat within PPP2RRB
SCA 17	—	Chorea, cognitive changes, psychosis, seizures[93]	CAG or CAA expansion within TBP
SCA 21	—	Cognitive changes, tremor[97,98]	Mutation within TMEM240

Clinical practice guidelines for PD genetic testing were last issued 10 years ago by the European Federation of Neurological Societies and were limited. Harbo and colleagues[99] recommended (1) LRRK2 full gene sequencing in AD familial cases, (2) LRRK2 G2019S testing in Ashkenazi Jewish or North African Berber Arabs with PD with or without a family history, and (3) PRKN, PINK1, and DJ-1 gene testing for families with recessive inheritance and/or in sporadic cases of early-onset PD. There has been reluctance on the part of the medical community to recommend genetic testing for PD to a broader population of patients because there was no clear benefit and it did not influence treatment. The recent emergence of targeted clinical trials for patients with PD who have GBA or LRRK2 mutations has influenced the risk-versus-benefit discussion toward more widespread testing and it is an appropriate time to reevaluate recommendations.

The authors are proposing that genetic testing be considered for PD for 2 reasons:

1. To divide this heterogeneous group of patients into subtypes to better understand the disease process and provide more specific clinical information regarding disease course
2. To provide patients the opportunity to participate in clinical trials based on their gene status

The intention here is to provide health care professionals with an approach to genetic testing in PD (**Fig. 1**), and, as more genetic risk factors are identified, readers may incorporate new information into the general construct provided. Genetic testing is addressed here for 3 separate categories of patients:

1. Affected individuals that are at high risk for a gene mutation
2. Affected individuals at low risk for a gene mutation

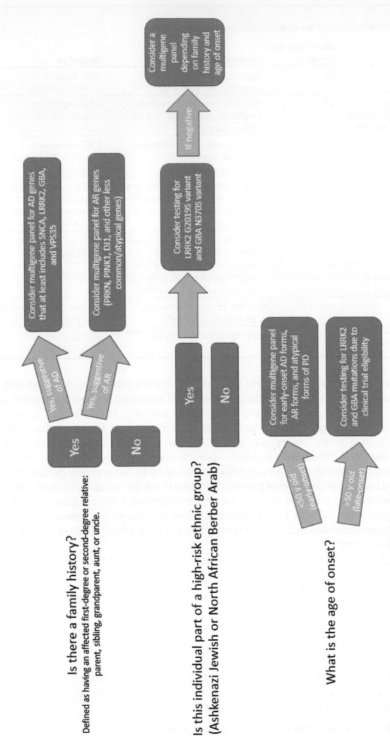

Fig. 1. PD genetic testing in an affected individual.

3. Unaffected individuals in the general population who decide to undergo genetic screening through DTC testing

Before genetic testing, clinicians should consider the patient's motivation and goals for testing and the implications of a positive or negative test result. Practical aspects of testing include:

1. Psychological impact of learning genetic information
2. Implications for family members
3. Eligibility for clinical trials
4. Medical record/insurance concerns
5. Possible guilt about transmitting a risk factor for a degenerative disease to children

It is important to keep in mind that patients may be hesitant about the inclusion of genetic information into the medical record because of potential consequences (real or perceived) for family members and concerns regarding insurance discrimination. Informed consent is the first and most important step in genetic testing. Often, this is not a decision made in a single visit, but may require a variable period of deliberation and dialogue with the practitioner/counselor before the patient makes the decision to proceed with testing.

Following informed consent, genetic testing should be strongly considered in individuals with any of the following risk factors:

1. Family history of PD (first-degree or second-degree relative affected)
2. Individuals of Ashkenazi Jewish or North African Berber Arab descent
3. Early-onset PD (before age 50 years)

Testing based on family history
Genetic testing for PD should ideally start with an affected individual. A family history should be performed, documenting parkinsonism, dementia, dystonia, ataxia, and related neurodegenerative diagnoses. If the family history is suggestive of AD inheritance, testing of *SNCA*, *LRRK2*, *GBA*, and other AD PD genes should be strongly considered. When the family history is suggestive of AR inheritance, testing for *PRKN*, *PINK1*, *DJ-1*, and other AR genes should be strongly considered. Many commercially available panels include AD, AR, and X-linked PD genes within the same test, which is helpful when the pattern of inheritance in the family is not straightforward.

Testing based on ethnicity
In individuals of Ashkenazi Jewish or North African Berber Arab descent, testing for the *LRRK2* G2019S and *GBA* N370S mutations should be strongly considered because of the high prevalence of these variants within these populations. If negative, a larger multigene panel that includes *LRRK2* and *GBA* full gene sequencing, as well as additional PD genes, may be considered.

Testing based on age of onset
In early-onset PD, testing for AR gene mutations (eg, *PRKN*, *PINK1*, *DJ-1*) and *GBA* should be strongly considered.

Testing in patients with sporadic Parkinson disease
Patients with PD with no family history, who are not Ashkenazi Jewish or North African Berber Arab, and have onset after age 50 years are much less likely to have a genetic component. However, testing may be considered for the 2 commonly occurring mutations for *LRRK2* and *GBA* because of the availability of clinical trials based on gene

status. Testing in this group of individuals with seemingly sporadic PD should only be ordered after a full discussion of the risks versus benefits and can be done through a health care professional or DTC testing. Many patients see DTC as advantageous and less threatening because the information is not placed into the medical record; however, there is more opportunity for clinical correlation and genetic counseling if they have testing through a medical professional.

Testing in unaffected individuals with no risk factors

The public is increasingly interested in learning about their genetic risk for a variety of disorders, and unaffected individuals with no risk factors for monogenic PD are undergoing DTC genetic screening. Testing may or may not be overseen by health professionals, and the information generated is often complex, requiring assistance with results interpretation. There is a risk of patients becoming distressed and/or confused by genetic testing information, and it is important to consider the impact of results before testing. Pretest counseling should be considered as a way to address psychosocial impact, insurance concerns, and other implications of genetic testing.

Genetic results need to be interpreted to determine clinical relevance. Available resources include genetic counseling in person or via telemedicine and online tools (National Society of Genetic Counselors Find a Genetic Counselor, Genetics Home Reference, OMIM, www.mdsgene.org, and GeneReviews). Results disclosure should include penetrance information, clinical trial eligibility, and information for at-risk family members. Identification of a mutation associated with PD does not guarantee that an individual will develop PD, and a negative result does not eliminate a genetic risk. Currently available DTC testing only assesses for 2 specific mutations, in *LRRK2* (G2019S) and *GBA* (N370S), therefore a negative result can be misleading.

SUMMARY

The genetics of PD is expanding at a rapid pace such that even at the time of this publication there will have been further advances. In addition, many of the genes involved in the pathogenesis of PD have yet to be discovered. Looking to the future, it is hoped that genetic testing for PD will be expanded to provide patients with a deeper understanding of their illness and provide them the opportunity to participate in the increasingly targeted therapeutic trials that are on the horizon.

REFERENCES

1. Hirsch L, Jette N, Frolkis A, et al. The incidence of Parkinson's Disease: a systematic review and meta-analysis. Neuroepidemiology 2016;46:292–300.
2. Diem-Zangerl A, Seppi K, Wenning GK, et al. Mortality in Parkinson's disease: a 20-year follow-up study. Mov Disord 2009;24:819–25.
3. Scott L, Dawson VL, Dawson TM. Trumping neurodegeneration: targeting common pathways regulated by autosomal recessive Parkinson's disease genes. Exp Neurol 2017;298:191–201.
4. Postuma R, Berg D, Stern M, et al. MDS clinical diagnostic criteria for Parkinson's disease. Mov Disord 2015;30:1591–9.
5. Ba F, Martin WRW. Dopamine transporter imaging as a diagnostic tool for parkinsonism and related disorders in clinical practice. Parkinsonism Relat Disord 2015;21:87–94.
6. Marshall VL, Reininger CB, Marquardt M, et al. Parkinson's disease is overdiagnosed clinically at baseline in diagnostically uncertain cases: a 3-year European multicenter study with repeat [^{123}I]FP-CIT SPECT. Mov Disord 2009;24:500–8.

7. Snow BJ, Tooyama EG, McGerr T, et al. Human positron emission tomographic ^{18}F-dopa studies correlate with dopamine cell counts and levels. Ann Neurol 1993;34:324–30.
8. Ibrahim N, Kusmirek J, Struck A, et al. The sensitivity and specificity of F-DOPA PET in a movement disorder clinic. Am J Nucl Med Mol Imaging 2016;6:102–9.
9. Pavese N, Brooks DJ. Imaging neurodegeneration in Parkinson's disease. Biochim Biophys Acta 2009;1792:722–9.
10. Kägi G, Bhatia KP, Tolosa E. The role of DAT-SPECT in movement disorders. J Neurol Neurosurg Psychiatry 2010;81:5–12.
11. Scherfler C, Schwarz J, Antonini A, et al. Role of DAT-SPECT in the diagnostic work up of Parkinsonism. Mov Disord 2007;22:1229–38.
12. Golbe LI, Di Lori G, Bonavita V, et al. A large kindred with autosomal dominant Parkinson's disease. Ann Neurol 1990;27:276–82.
13. Polymeropoulos MH, Lavedan C, Leroy E, et al. Mutation in the alpha-synuclein gene identified in families with Parkinson's disease. Science 1997;27:2045–7.
14. Singleton A, Farrer M, Johnson J, et al. α-Synuclein locus triplication causes parkinson's disease. Science 2003;302:841.
15. Jankovic J, Goodman I, Safirstein B, et al. Safety and tolerability of multiple ascending doses of PRX002/RG7935, and anti-synuclein monoclonal antibody, in patients with Parkinson disease: a randomized clinical trial. JAMA Neurol 2018;75:1206–14.
16. Várkonyi J, Rosenbaum H, Bauman N, et al. Gaucher disease associated with parkinsonism: four further case reports. Am J Med Genet A 2003;116A:348–51.
17. Lwin A, Orvisky E, Goker-Alpan O, et al. Glucocerebrosidase mutations in subjects with parkinsonism. Mol Genet Metab 2004;81:70–3.
18. Rosenbloom B, Balwani M, Bronstein J, et al. The incidence of Parkinsonism in patients with type 1 Gaucher disease: data from the ICGG Gaucher registry. Blood Cell Mol Dis 2011;46:95–102.
19. Farlow J. Parkinson disease overview. Ncbi.nlm.nih.gov. 2004. Available at: https://www.ncbi.nlm.nih.gov/books/NBK1223/. Accessed January 12, 2019.
20. Wirdefeldt K, Gatz M, Reynolds CA, et al. Heritability of Parkinson disease in Swedish twins: a longitudinal study. Neurobiol Aging 2011;32:1923.e1-8.
21. Deng H, Peng W, Jankovic J. The genetics of Parkinson disease. Ageing Res Rev 2018;42:72–85.
22. Hernandez D, Reed X, Singleton A. Genetics in Parkinson disease: mendelian vs. non-Mendelian inheritance. J Neurochem 2016;139:59–74.
23. Trinh J, Guella I, Farrer M. Disease penetrance of late-onset parkinsonism: a meta-analysis. JAMA Neurol 2014;71(12):1535–9.
24. Marras C, Lang A, van de Warrenburg BP, et al. Nomenclature of genetic movement disorders: Recommendations of the international Parkinson and movement disorder society task force. Mov Disord 2016;31:436–57.
25. Domingo A, Klein C. Genetics of Parkinson disease. Handbk Clin Neurol 2018; 147:211–27.
26. SNCA gene: National Library of Medicine (US). Genetics home reference. Bethesda (MD). 2018. Available at: https://ghr.nlm.nih.gov/gene/SNCA. Accessed February 8 2019.
27. Bardien S, Lesage S, Brice A, et al. Genetic characteristics of leucine-rich repeat kinase 2 (LRRK2) associated Parkinson's disease. Parkinsonism Relat Disord 2011;17:501–8.
28. Funayama M, Hasegawa K, Kowa H, et al. A new locus for Parkinson's disease (PARK8) maps to chromosome 12p11.2-q13.1. Ann Neurol 2002;51:296–301.

29. Zimprich A, Biskup S, Leitner P, et al. Mutations in LRRK2 cause autosomal dominant parkinsonism with pleomorphic pathology. Neuron 2004;44:601–7.

30. Henry AG, Aghamohammadzadeh S, Samaroo H, et al. Pathogenic LRRK2 mutations, through increased kinase activity, produce enlarged lysosomes with reduced degradative capacity and increase ATP13A2 expression. Hum Mol Genet 2015;24:6013–28.

31. Healy DG, Falchi M, O'Sullivan SS, et al. International LRRK2 Consortium. Phenotype, genotype, and worldwide genetic penetrance of LRRK2-associated Parkinson's disease: a case-control study. Lancet Neurol 2008;7:583–90.

32. Nichols WC, Pankratz N, Hernandez D, et al. Genetic screening for a single common LRRK2 mutation in familial Parkinson's disease. Lancet 2005;365:410–2.

33. Ozelius LJ, Senthil G, Saunders-Pullman R, et al. LRRK2 G2019S as a cause of Parkinson's disease in Ashkenazi Jews. N Engl J Med 2006;354:424–5.

34. Lesage S, Dürr A, Tazier M, et al. *LRRK2* G2019S as a cause of Parkinson's disease in North African Arabs. N Engl J Med 2006;354:422–3.

35. Hulihan MM, Ishihara-Paul L, Kachergus J, et al. LRRK2 Gly2019Ser penetrance in Arab-Berber patients from Tunisia: a case-control genetic study. Lancet Neurol 2008;7:591–4.

36. Lee AJ, Wang Y, Alcalay RN, et al. Penetrance estimate of LRRK2 p.G2019S mutation in individuals of non-Ashkenazi Jewish ancestry. Mov Disord 2017;32: 1432–8.

37. Ruiz-Martínez J, Gorostidi A, Ibañez B, et al. Penetrance in Parkinson's disease related to the *LRRK2* R1441G mutation in the Basque country (Spain). Mov Disord 2010;25:2340–5.

38. Farrer MJ, Stone JT, Lin CH, et al. Lrrk2 G2385R is an ancestral risk factor for Parkinson's disease in Asia. Parkinsonism Relat Disord 2007;13:89–92.

39. Sidransky E, Nalls MA, Aasly JO, et al. Multicenter analysis of glucocerebrosidase mutations in Parkinson's disease. N Engl J Med 2009;361:1651–61.

40. Gan-Or Z, Amshalom I, Kilarski LL, et al. Differential effects of severe vs mild GBA mutations on Parkinson disease. Neurology 2015;84:880–7.

41. Alcalay RN, Dinur T, Quinn T, et al. Comparison of Parkinson risk in Ashkenazi Jewish patients with Gaucher disease and GBA heterozygotes. JAMA Neurol 2014;71:752–7.

42. Malek N, Weil RS, Bresner C, et al. Features of GBA-associated Parkinson's disease at presentation in the UK Tracking Parkinson's study. J Neurol Neurosurg Psychiatry 2018;89:702–9.

43. Setó-Salvia N, Pagonabarraga J, Houlden H, et al. Glucocerebrosidase mutations confer a greater risk of dementia during Parkinson's disease course. Mov Disord 2012;27:393–9.

44. Leroy E, Boyer R, Auburger G, et al. The ubiquitin pathway in Parkinson's disease. Nature 1998;395:451–2.

45. Vilarino-Guell C, Wider C, Ross OA, et al. VPS35 mutations in Parkinson disease. Am J Hum Genet 2011;89:162–7 [Note: Erratum: Am J Hum Genet 2011;89: 347 only].

46. Zimprich A, Benet-Pages A, Struhal W, et al. A mutation in VPS35 encoding a subunit of the retromer complex, causes late-onset Parkinson disease. Am J Hum Genet 2011;89:168–75.

47. Chartier-Harlin MC, Dachsel JC, Vilarino-Guell C, et al. Translation initiator EIF4G1 mutations in familial Parkinson disease. Am J Hum Genet 2011;89:398–406.

48. Suzuki Y, Imai Y, Nakayama H, et al. A serine protease, HtrA2, is released from the mitochondria and interacts with XIAP, inducing cell death. Mol Cell 2001;8: 613–21.

49. Strauss KM, Martins LM, Plun-Favreau H, et al. Loss of function mutations in the gene encoding Omi/HtrA2 in Parkinson's disease. Hum Mol Genet 2005;14: 2099–111.

50. Aras S, Oleg P, Sommer N, et al. Oxygen-dependent expression of cytochrome *c* oxidase subunit 4-2 gene expression is mediated by transcription factors RBPJ, CXXC5 and CHCHD2. Nucleic Acids Res 2013;41:2255–66.

51. Funayama M, Ohe K, Amo T, et al. CHCHD2 mutations in autosomal dominant late-onset Parkinson's disease: a genome-wide linkage and sequencing study. Lancet Neurol 2015;14:274–82.

52. Vilarino-Guell C, Rajput A, Milnerwood AJ, et al. DNAJC13 mutations in Parkinson disease. Hum Mol Genet 2014;23:1794–801.

53. Kim C, Alcalay R. Genetic forms of Parkinson's disease. Semin Neurol 2017;37: 135–46.

54. Nardin A, Schrepfer E, Ziviani E. Counteracting PINK/Parkin deficiency in the activation of mitophagy: a potential therapeutic intervention for Parkinson's disease. Curr Neuropharmacol 2016;14:250–9.

55. Lücking C, Dürr A, Bonifati V, et al. Association between early-onset Parkinson's Disease and mutations in the *PARKIN* gene. N Engl J Med 2000;342:1560–7.

56. Hoenicka J, Vidal L, Morales B, et al. Molecular findings in familial Parkinson disease in Spain. Arch Neurol 2002;59:966–70.

57. Valente EM, Abou-Sleiman PM, Caputo V, et al. Hereditary early-onset Parkinson's Disease caused by mutations in PINK1. Science 2004;304:1158–60.

58. Durcan TM, Fon EA. The three 'P's of mitophagy: PARKIN, PINK1, and post-translational modifications. Genes Dev 2015;29:989–99.

59. Valente EM, Salvi S, Ialongo T, et al. PINK1 mutations are associated with sporadic early-onset parkinsonism. Ann Neurol 2004;56:335–41.

60. Xu J, Zhong N, Wang H, et al. The Parkinson's disease-associated DJ-1 protein is a transcriptional co-activator that protects against neuronal apoptosis. Hum Mol Genet 2005;14:1231–41.

61. Irrcher I, Aleyasin H, Seifert EL, et al. Loss of Parkinson's disease-linked gene DJ-1 perturbs mitochondrial dynamics. Hum Mol Genet 2010;19:3734–46.

62. Park JS, Blair NF, Sue CM. The role of ATP13A2 in Parkinson's Disease: clinical phenotypes and molecular mechanisms. Mov Disord 2015;30:770–9.

63. Ho M, Ou C, Chan YR, et al. The utility F-box for protein destruction. Cell Mol Life Sci 2008;65:1977–2000.

64. Zhou ZD, Xie SP, Sathiyamoorthy S, et al. F-box protein 7 mutations promote protein aggregation in mitochondria and inhibit mitophagy. Hum Mol Genet 2015;24: 6314–30.

65. Di Fonzo A, Dekker MCJ, Baruzzi A, et al. *FBXO7* mutations cause autosomal recessive, early-onset parkinsonian-pyramidal syndrome. Neurology 2009;72: 240–5.

66. Kurian MA, Zhen J, Cheng SY, et al. Homozygous loss-of-function mutations in the gene encoding the dopamine transporter are associated with infantile parkinsonism-dystonia. J Clin Invest 2009;119:1595–603.

67. Kurian MA, Yan L, Zhen J, et al. Clinical and molecular characterization of hereditary dopamine transporter deficiency syndrome: an observational cohort and experimental study. Lancet Neurol 2010;10:54–62.

68. Kurian MA. SLC6A3-related dopamine transporter deficiency syndrome. Seattle, WA: Gene Reviews; 2017. Available at: https://www.ncbi.nlm.nih.gov/books/NBK442323/. Accessed January 05, 2019.

69. Paisan-Ruiz C, Bhatia KP, Li A, et al. Characterization of *PLA2G6* as a locus for dystonia-parkinsonism. Ann Neurol 2009;65:19–23.

70. Edvardson S, Cimmamon Y, Ta-Shma A, et al. A deleterious mutation in *DNAJC6* encoding the neuronal-specific clathrin-uncoating co-chaperone auxilin, is associated with juvenile parkinsonism. PLoS One 2012;7:e36458. Available at: www.plosone.org. Accessed January 2, 2019.

71. Elsayed LEO, Drouet V, Usenko T, et al. A novel nonsense mutation in DNAJC6 expands the phenotype of autosomal-recessive juvenile-onset Parkinson's disease. Ann Neurol 2016;79:35–8.

72. Koroglu C, Baysal L, Cetinkaya M, et al. DNAJC is responsible for juvenile parkinsonism with phenotypic variability. Parkinsonism Relat Disord 2013;19:320–4.

73. Olgiati S, Quadri M, Fang M, et al. *DNAJC6* mutations associated with early-onset Parkinson's Disease. Ann Neurol 2016;79:244–56.

74. Krebs C, Karkheiran S, Powell JC, et al. The sac1 domain of *SYNJ1* identified mutated in a family with early-onset progressive parkinsonism with generalized seizures. Hum Mutat 2013;34:1200–7.

75. Quadri M, Fang M, Picillo M, et al. Mutation in the *SYNJ1* gene associated with autosomal recessive, early-onset parkinsonism. Hum Mutat 2013;34:1208–15.

76. Lesage S, Drouet V, Majounie E, et al. Loss of VPS13C function in autosomal-recessive parkinsonism causes mitochondrial dysfunction and increases PINK1/Parkin-dependent mitophagy. Am J Hum Genet 2016;98:500–13.

77. National Library of Medicine (US). X-linked dystonia-parkinsonism: genetic home reference 2008. National Institutes of Health. Bethesda (MD). Available at: https://ghr.nlm.nih.gov/gene/SNCA. Accessed February 5 2019.

78. Wijemanne S, Jankovic J. Dopa-responsive dystonia-clinical and genetic heterogeneity. Nat Rev Neurol 2015;11:414–24.

79. Jacquemont S, Hagerman R, Leehey M, et al. Fragile X premutation tremor/ataxia syndrome: molecular, clinical, and neuroimaging correlates. Am J Hum Genet 2003;74:869–78.

80. Rousseau F, Rouillard P, Morel ML, et al. Prevalence of carriers of premutation-size alleles of the FMRI gene–and implications for the population genetics of the fragile X syndrome. Am J Hum Genet 1995;57:1006–18.

81. Dombrowski C, Lévesque S, Morel ML, et al. Premutation and intermediate-size *FMR1* alleles in 10 572 males from the general population: loss of an AGG interruption is a late event in the generation of fragile X syndrome alleles. Hum Mol Genet 2002;11:371–8.

82. Hagerman RJ, Leehey M, Heinrichs W, et al. Intention tremor, parkinsonism, and generalized brain atrophy in male carriers of fragile X. Neurology 2001;57:127–30.

83. Juncos JL, Lazarus JT, Graves-Allen E, et al. New clinical findings in the fragile X-associated tremor ataxia syndrome (FXTAS). Neurogenetics 2011;12:123–35.

84. Niu YQ, Yang JC, Hall D, et al. Parkinsonism in fragile X-associated tremor/ataxia syndrome (FXTAS): Revisited. Parkinsonism Relat Disord 2014;20:456–9.

85. Jacquemont S, Hagerman RJ, Leehey MA, et al. Penetrance of the Fragile X–associated tremor/ataxia syndrome in a premutation carrier population. JAMA 2004;29:460–9.

86. Fraint A, Padmaja V, Aimee S, et al. New observations in the fragile X-associated tremor/ataxia syndrome (FXTAS) phenotype. Front Genet 2014;5:365.

87. Apartis E, Blancher A, Meissner WG, et al. FXTAS new insights and the need for revised diagnostic criteria. Neurology 2012;79:1898–907.
88. Park H, Kim HJ, Jeon BS. Parkinsonism in spinocerebellar ataxia. Biomed Res Int 2015;ID 125273:1–11.
89. Cancel G, Dürr A, Didierjean O, et al. Molecular and clinical correlations in spinocerebellar ataxia 2: a study of 32 families. Hum Mol Genet 1997;6:709–15.
90. Gwinn-Hardy K, Singleton A, O'Suilleabhain p, et al. Spinocerebellar ataxia type 3 phenotypically resembling Parkinson disease in a black family. Arch Neurol 2001; 58:296–9.
91. Tuite PJ, Rogaeva A, St George-Hyslop PH, et al. Dopa-responsive parkinsonism phenotype of Machado-Joseph Disease: confirmation of 14q CAG expansion. Ann Neurol 1995;38:684–7.
92. Gomez C, Thompson R, Gammack JT, et al. Spinocerebellar ataxia type 6: gaze-evoked and vertical nystagmus, Purkinje cell degeneration, and variable age of onset. Ann Neurol 1997;42:933–50.
93. Schöls L, Bauer P, Schmidt T, et al. Autosomal dominant cerebellar ataxias: clinical features, genetics, and pathogenesis. Lancet Neurol 2004;3:291–304.
94. Ayhan F, Ikeda Y, Dalton JC, et al. Spinocerebellar ataxia type 8. Seattle, WA: Gene Reviews; 2001. Available at: https://www.ncbi.nlm.nih.gov/books/NBK1268. Accessed January 9, 2019.
95. O'Hearn E, Holmes SE, Calvert PC, et al. SCA-12: tremor with cerebellar and cortical atrophy is associated with a CAG repeat expansion. Neurology 2001; 56:299–303.
96. Holmes SE, O'Hearn E, Roos CA, et al. SCA12: an unusual mutation leads to an unusual spinocerebellar ataxia. Brain Res Bull 2001;56:397–403.
97. Delplanque J, Devos D, Huin V, et al. TMEM240 mutations cause spinocerebellar ataxia 21 with mental retardation and severe cognitive impairment. Brain 2014; 137:2657–63.
98. Devos D, Schraen-Maschke S, Vuillaume I, et al. Clinical features and genetic analysis of a new form of spinocerebellar ataxia. Neurology 2001;56:234–8.
99. Harbo HF, Finsterer J, Baets J, et al. EFNS guidelines on the molecular diagnosis of neurogenetic disorders: general issues, Huntington's disease, Parkinson's disease and dystonias. Eur J Neurol 2009;16:777–85.

Population Whole Exome Screening

Primary Care Provider Attitudes About Preparedness, Information Avoidance, and Nudging

Patrick R. Heck, PhD[a,b], Michelle N. Meyer, PhD, JD[b,c],*

KEYWORDS

- Information avoidance • Nudge • Ethics • Whole exome sequencing
- Personalized medicine • Genetics • Genomics • Population screening

KEY POINTS

- Health systems can successfully incorporate genomics into primary care despite limited provider training and confidence in their ability to answer patients' questions about their risk for inherited conditions.
- Compared to laypeople (N = 1605), primary care providers (N = 426) reported strong but varied preferences to seek or receive genetic health information about themselves.
- Providers largely supported population genomic screening and typically reported willingness to get screened themselves, although some raised concerns about insurance discrimination, lack of patient and provider education, and data privacy.
- A large majority of primary care providers judged a hypothetical patient's decision to undergo clinical whole-exome sequencing favorably relative to a similar patient's decision not to undergo such testing.
- These providers, a small sample of genetics specialists, and a small sample of patients held mixed attitudes toward 2 nudges designed to increase uptake for cascade testing among at-risk relatives of variant-positive patients.

INTRODUCTION

Geisinger is a large, physician-led, integrated health system serving 4.2 million residents in central and northeast Pennsylvania and southern New Jersey. Fourteen

Disclosure Statement: The authors have nothing to disclose.
[a] Autism & Developmental Medicine Institute, Geisinger, 120 Hamm Drive, M-C 60-36, Lewisburg, PA 17827, USA; [b] Center for Translational Bioethics and Health Care Policy, Geisinger, Danville, PA 17822, USA; [c] Behavioral Insights Team, Steele Institute for Health Innovation, Geisinger, 100 North Academy Avenue, M-C 30-57, Danville, PA 17822, USA
* Corresponding author.
E-mail address: michellenmeyer@gmail.com
twitter: @P_HECK (P.R.H.); @MICHELLENMEYER (M.N.M.)

hospitals and 216 primary and specialty clinics, including 106 community-based primary care clinics, comprise Geisinger's 2-state network. About one-third of Geisinger patients are insured by the provider-owned Geisinger Health Plan.

In the early 2000s, Geisinger leadership began discussing a genomics core to support its research strategic plan of precision health, which led to the development of an unselected biobank, MyCode, in 2007.[1] Patients approached in primary and specialty clinics give broad, opt-in consent to have their DNA and electronic health records used in discovery research. Beginning in 2014, through a partnership with Regeneron Genetics Center, a wholly owned subsidiary of Regeneron Pharmaceuticals, Inc., Geisinger began conducting whole exome sequencing (WES) of MyCode samples.[2] Geisinger made an institutional decision to return clinically actionable results of this WES to patient-participants and their primary care physicians and to place such information in the patient's electronic health record where it can guide preventive care according to clinical guidelines.[3] The protocol and consent form for MyCode—by then called the MyCode Community Health Initiative—were modified to allow for this, and by May of 2015, what is now called the MyCode Genomic Screening and Counseling (GSC) Program began. Through the GSC Program, patient-participant exomes are screened for pathogenic or likely pathogenic variants in an initial list of 76 genes (now 80 genes, with the addition of 5 and removal of 1) associated with preventable and/or treatable monogenic conditions. This list includes but builds on the American College of Medical Genetics and Genomics list of reportable secondary findings. A variant-positive MyCode research result is sent to a Clinical Laboratory Improvement Amendment-certified laboratory for confirmation before being returned to the patient and his or her primary care physician. The GSC Program also facilitates condition-specific clinical evaluations and cascade testing of at-risk relatives.[4]

As of August 2019, more than 250,000 patients have been consented to MyCode, more than 92,000 of whom have had their whole exomes sequenced. To date, 1073 clinically confirmed results from 45 genes have been reported to 1068 patients and their primary care physicians and entered into the electronic health record.[5] About one-half of these clinical results are for Centers for Disease Control and Prevention tier 1 conditions: hereditary breast and ovarian cancer, familial hypercholesterolemia, and Lynch syndrome.[6] The vast majority of the remaining results are mutations that cause cardiovascular disease, other cancers, or hereditary hemochromatosis.[7] In many cases, variant-positive patients were currently healthy, unaware of their increased risk, and would not have qualified by either personal or family history for clinical testing.[8,9]

In May of 2018, then-Geisinger CEO David Feinberg announced that Geisinger would begin offering clinical WES to patients in primary care clinics.[10] Although the program has launched in 2 clinics initially—the Internal Medicine Clinic at Geisinger Medical Center in Danville, Pennsylvania, and at the Kistler Clinic in Wilkes-Barre, Pennsylvania, with the Geisinger Health Plan covering the cost for the first 1000 patients—the intention is for clinical WES eventually to be offered to all Geisinger patients seen in primary care clinics. The early MyCode experience suggests that about 3.5% of patients will have pathogenic or likely pathogenic variants that meet criteria for clinical action,[2] although that number is expected to increase to as many as 10% to 15% of patients as more is learned about the effect of different genetic variants on a variety of health conditions.[11] To date, the clinical WES program has identified 14 variant-positive patients; in several of these cases, the patient's increased risk constituted new information for both patient and provider.

Given its success with MyCode and its innovative clinical WES program, Geisinger is frequently described as leading the way in integrating genomics into primary care[12] and participates in national conversations about the same.[13] Geisinger's experience raises several questions for other health systems interested in incorporating genomics into clinical care. In their systematic review of the literature exploring the role of primary care in genetic services, Emery and colleagues[14] found that although primary care providers (PCPs) generally supported patient access to genetic services for both Mendelian and multifactorial disease, including carrier, predictive, and prenatal testing, most had limited knowledge of medical genetics; preferred to limit their own role in such services to gatekeeping, family history taking, and supportive counseling; and even lacked confidence in their ability to take a detailed family history. Lack of provider preparedness is frequently cited as an obstacle to integrating genomics into medical care, including in commentaries that discuss Geisinger's research and clinical genomic programs.[10] Rather than relying on provider expertise in genomics, Geisinger provides primary care physicians whose patient tests variant-positive (whether through MyCode or clinical WES) with a "just-in-time," gene-specific educational module.

This article reviews the results of prior survey studies of PCP characteristics of relevance to genomic medicine and report results of our own survey of Geisinger PCPs—primary care physicians and clinic-based nurse practitioners (NPs), physician assistants (PAs), and nurses. It also explores for the first time in the literature 2 broad sets of questions that will become important as genomic medicine progresses. First, how do providers perceive patients who decline population genomic screening? Would providers themselves choose to pursue or avoid such information? Second, do PCPs support efforts to nudge at-risk relatives identified as the result of population screening to get genomic counseling and testing? Do the views of PCPs differ from those of laypersons or genetic counselors?

METHODS AND SAMPLE

Between September 24 and October 8, 2018, we anonymously surveyed all PCPs throughout Geisinger's Pennsylvania catchment area (N = 426 complete responses, 9.4% response rate). Our 35-item questionnaire asked about several topics related to population genetic screening, including attitudes toward hypothetical information-avoidant patients and nudges to encourage the uptake of genomic counseling and testing for patients at risk for actionable variants. We also asked about participants' attitudes toward randomized evaluation versus universal implementation of medical practices, reported elsewhere.[15] We included nurses in our survey because, although they are important to the integration of genomics into medicine,[16–18] their attitudes are rarely elicited in surveys. Participation was incentivized by offering a chance to win one of eight $50 Amazon gift cards. Respondents were recruited by an email sent by the medical director of one of the 2 clinics where clinical WES screening is active. The email explained that the purpose of the survey was to study attitudes toward Geisinger's new clinical WES program and patients who are offered this service, and reminded participants that if they do not work in 1 of the 2 clinics currently offering this test, they can expect to be in this position in the near future as the test rolls out across the system. **Table 1** displays the sample characteristics in terms of position, years spent working at Geisinger, and years spent working in medicine. We did not collect typical demographic information (ie, age, sex, and race/ethnicity) during this survey to ensure respondents' anonymity.

Table 1
Clinician education and experience with genetic screening

Choice Options	Percentage of Sample
Position	
Physician	36.6
PA	6.1
NP	6.1
Nurse	50.5
Other	0.7
Years at Geisinger	
<1	7.3
1–2	20.0
3–5	19.5
6–10	19.2
>10	34.0
Years in medicine	
<1	0.9
1–2	4.9
3–5	14.3
6–10	12.2
>10	67.6

CHARACTERISTICS OF GEISINGER PRIMARY CARE PROVIDERS
Training and Education in Genetics

A large survey (N = 3686) of primary care physicians in western Europe found that 19% of general practitioners, and 13% of obstetrician/gynecologist specialists and 12% of pediatricians working in a primary care setting, reported having no genetics training.[19] In our survey, we found only a slightly lower rate of primary care physicians at Geisinger who reported no genetics training (8%). Of those respondents who did report some form of genetics training, the nature of that training (**Table 2**) was similar to that reported in some other samples. For instance, a prior survey of predominantly primary care physicians found that 29% reported medical school training in genetics (vs 45% in our sample), 35% reported training during their residency (vs 29%), and 66% reported training via Continuing Medical Education (CME) courses (vs 22%).[20] In a survey of 1008 Italian physicians, only a minority reported having had exposure to cancer genetic testing during their graduate (20%) or postgraduate (21%) training.[21] In a US national survey (N = 1120), 61% of primary care physicians reported genetics training in medical school (vs 45% in our sample) and 47% reporting training via CME courses (vs 22%).[22] A recent survey of nurses found that only 30% reported having taken a genetics course since licensure, and 94% reported interest in learning more about genomics.[23] Compared with previous work, our survey found similar rates of genetics training in professional schools and postgraduate education, but lower reported rates of CME.

Genetic Test Ordering and Referral and Predictors of These Behaviors

Most previous surveys have explored self-reported ordering and referral behavior in the cancer genetics context. A survey of family practitioner and specialist physicians (N = 1500) found that only 25% reported having ordered a *BRCA* test within the

Table 2
Clinician education and experience with genetic screening

Options	% of Sample (N = 426)	% of Physicians (n = 156)	% of PAs/NPs (n = 52)	% of Nurses (n = 215)
Training in genetics				
Undergraduate	32	48	50	16
Professional school	21	45	21	4
Postgraduate	12	29	10	1
CME	18	22	35	12
Independent study	17	31	23	7
None of these	39	8	17	66
Professional experience with genetic screening				
Ordered a genetic test	19	41	31	1
Returned a genetic result	16	32	23	2
Referred a patient for testing	28	59	35	4
Discussed or ordered WES	4	8	0	0
None of these	65	30	52	94
Personal experience with genetic screening				
DTC test for ancestry	10	13	8	8
DTC test for health	2	4	0	1
Clinical genetic testing	10	9	8	10
Participated in Biobank research	35	31	46	34
Had clinical WES screening	2	4	0	0
None of these	55	54	46	58

For all variables, participants were allowed to select more than one option.
Abbreviation: DTC, direct to consumer.

previous year.[24] In a 2010 survey, 25% to 67% (depending on the particular test) of Oregon PCP respondents (physicians, NPs, and PAs) reported ordering *BRCA* or Lynch syndrome tests in the previous year, and 56% to 68% reported having referred a patient for testing.[25] A survey of 475 primary care physicians practicing in southeastern Pennsylvania and southern New Jersey (included in Geisinger's catchment area) found that 37% reported having either ordered or referred patients for any cancer susceptibility testing in the previous year.[26] A survey of 254 primary care physicians found that 21% had referred patients for cancer genetic testing in the prior year.[27] A national survey of primary care physicians (N = 1120) found that 60% had ever ordered any genetic test, 74% had ever referred a patient for any genetic testing, and 81% had at least 1 experience with ordering or referral.[22]

Our survey asked Geisinger PCPs whether they had ordered or referred for any genetic test in the previous year. Sifri et al.[26] found that ordering/referral was positively associated with working in an integrated health system, like Geisinger. Nevertheless, only 35% of Geisinger PCPs reported having direct professional experience with genetic medicine (70% of physicians, 48% of PAs and NPs, and 6% of nurses), either by referring, ordering, returning a genetic result, or discussing or ordering WES testing as part of their job. More PCPs had referred (28%) than ordered (19%), and only a small number had returned a genetic result to a patient (16%) or discussed or ordered WES (4%).

Shields and colleagues[22] found that factors associated with having ever ordered a genetic test included having had genetics training in medical school, having had such training via CME courses, and self-reported feeling of preparedness to counsel patients considering a genetic test—but not self-reported confidence in interpreting genetic test results. Only having had clinical genetics training via CME courses was associated with having ever referred a patient for genetic testing. Ordering has also been associated with having been in practice more than 10 years (27.5% vs 21.7%).[24] A survey of 220 internists from 2 academic medical centers found that 41% rated their knowledge of genetics, and 42% rated their knowledge of genetic testing guidelines, to be very or somewhat poor.[28] Yet, 26% of these internists had ordered testing, despite reporting that they were somewhat or very uncomfortable ordering or referring patients for testing. Similarly, 40% had ordered tests despite reporting that they were somewhat or very uncomfortable counseling patients on genetic testing. In our survey, after excluding nurses from analyses (leaving 211 responses), we explored what other variables were associated with having ordered a genetic test for a patient. Bivariate correlations revealed several notable positive relationships with having ordered a genetic test, including:

- How many sources of training a participant reported having ($r = 0.27$; $P<.001$)
- Having returned a result to a patient ($r = 0.64$; $P<.001$)
- Having referred a patient for a genetic test ($r = 0.35$; $P<.001$)
- Increased reported comfort answering patients' questions about their risk for inherited conditions ($r = 0.23$; $P<.001$)

Personal Experience with Genetics and Genomics

Interestingly, our sample of providers reported a breadth of personal experience with genetic testing: 45% of participants reported some form of personal experience, including (among others) purchasing direct-to-consumer testing, participating as a subject in genetics-related research (such as MyCode), or getting clinical genetic testing themselves (see **Table 2**). Across the entire sample (N = 426), we observed a small correlation between having had some form of genetic test and having ordered, referred, or returned a genetic result to a patient ($r = 0.12$; $P = .013$), suggesting that clinicians' personal attitudes toward or experience with genetic screening may not be fully independent from their professional recommendations.

Primary Care Provider Comfort Answering Patient Questions About Inherited Risk

A persistent finding of previous surveys is that although PCPs support the integration of genetics/omics into primary care, they do not feel confident in their knowledge of genetics. For instance, in a survey of academic family physicians in the United States and Canada (N = 1404), 72% of respondents felt that genetic testing was somewhat or very valuable in the primary care setting. Yet 54% reported feeling that they were not knowledgeable about currently available genetic tests they could use in practice and an additional 43% felt only somewhat knowledgeable.[29] A large survey of Italian physicians found that 80% viewed their knowledge of appropriate genetic testing for cancer to be inadequate and 94% thought their knowledge on this front should be improved.[21] A survey of 220 internists from 2 prominent US academic medical centers where respondents had "innumerable opportunities for continuing medical education" found that most nevertheless rated their knowledge of genetics (74%) and genetic testing guidelines (87%) as very or somewhat poor.[28] A survey of nurses found that most (68%) believed that genomics is very important to nursing practice, but 57% felt that their understanding of basic genomics was fair or poor (supported by 60%

incorrectly reporting that heart disease and diabetes are caused by a single gene variant).[16] And in a survey of primary care physicians, NPs, and PAs (N = 361), the vast majority of respondents reported being not at all (31%) or only somewhat (53%) confident in their personal knowledge of medical genetics relevant to breast, ovarian, and colorectal cancers.[25]

Perhaps as an understandable result of this perceived (and often objectively verified) lack of knowledge, PCPs consistently report low confidence in their ability to play a role in integrating genetics/omics into primary care. For instance, a large survey (N = 3686) of primary care physicians in France, Germany, the Netherlands, Sweden, and the UK found that 44.2% were not confident in their ability to carry out basic medical genetic tasks, 36.5% were somewhat confident, and only 19.3% were confident or very confident.[19] A survey of Scottish general practitioners found that the majority reported feeling only a little or not at all confident in calculating the risks associated with a family risk of cancer (95%) and counseling patients on their cancer risk (77%). Only a minority of respondents reported feeling confident or very confident, even with respect to those roles that most respondents embraced as properly within the scope of their practice: taking a detailed family history (39%), knowing which patients to refer to a cancer genetics clinic (27%), and discussing the need for mammography or colonoscopy screening with patients (33%).[30]

To gain insight into clinicians' level of comfort in interacting with patients on genomics-related topics, we asked, "How comfortable are you with answering patients' questions about their risk for inherited conditions?" (options ranging from 1 [not at all] to 5 [extremely] with a midpoint of 3 [moderately]). We found that clinicians reported being on average only just above somewhat comfortable answering patient questions about inherited risk (mean = 2.07; SD = 0.95). Unsurprisingly, nurses reported less comfort in this area (mean, 1.84; SD = 0.91) than prescribing clinicians (hereafter, "prescribers," to include physicians, PAs, and NPs) (mean = 2.33; SD = 0.91), $t(421) = 5.53$, $P<.001$, with a medium effect size in standard deviation units, $d = 0.54$ (**Fig. 1**). Few clinicians among our entire sample (no more than 7.4%) reported being either very or extremely comfortable discussing inherited risk with patients.

Previous studies have found that low confidence in carrying out basic medical genetic tasks was associated with less exposure to medical genetics training and education.[19] Perceived competence in providing health care to patients related to genetics and genomics was not associated with more recent training or with the number of genetic tests ordered annually.[31] A survey of 254 Alabama primary care physicians found that those in practice 10 years or less were more confident than were those practicing more than 20 years in explaining genetic test results to patients and in tailoring recommendations for screening.[27] Across our entire sample, we observed an encouraging positive relationship between the measure of comfort discussing genomics with patients and whether participants had any formal training in genetics ($r = 0.36$; $P<.001$), or professional experience with genetic testing ($r = 0.31$; $P<.001$). However, comfort level was not significantly associated with how long a participant had been working in medicine ($r = -0.08$; $P = .10$) or at Geisinger ($r = -0.07$; $P = .15$).

PROVIDER AND LAY ATTITUDES RELATED TO POPULATION GENOMIC SCREENING
Primary Care Provider Perceptions of Patients Who Seek or Avoid Genetic Health Information

We elicited PCP respondents' perceptions of hypothetical patients who choose to participate in or avoid Geisinger's new, free, clinical WES program (reported in

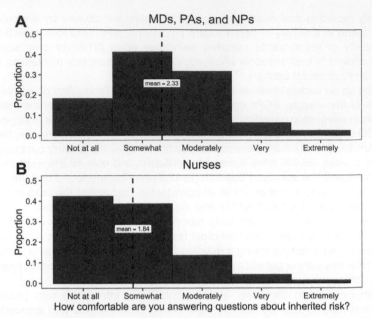

Fig. 1. Clinicians' reported level of comfort answering patients' questions about inherited risk. (*A*) Results for prescribers. (*B*) Results for nurses.

detail elsewhere[32]). PCPs gave more favorable ratings of a patient's traits and characteristics (ie, how intelligent, trustworthy, irrational, and principled, among other items, the patient is) when this patient chose to participate in the program than when he or she chose not to participate. Clinicians reported feeling greater empathy and sympathy for hypothetical patients who decided to enroll in the WES program, and evaluated enrollment as the right choice to a much greater extent than choosing not to enroll.

In addition to eliciting providers' attitudes toward patients in actionable scenarios (much like Geisinger's clinical WES program), we also asked some participants to assess a hypothetical patient who chose to enroll in a hypothetical future program that would return clinically nonactionable genetic health information, such as *APOE* genotype, which predicts risk for Alzheimer disease. Here, providers' evaluations did not differ between information-seeking and information-avoidant targets; PCPs' attitudes toward patients who sought and who avoided these results were extremely similar, and whether the hypothetical patient chose to pursue this information or not had no bearing on providers' judgments of whether the hypothetical patient made the right choice in this context. This finding is not especially surprising. Prior studies have found that physicians have expressed reluctance to discuss genetic risk with patients if an effective treatment or intervention is not available.[33] For instance, in a survey of community-based physicians treating patients with Alzheimer disease (N = 110), only 39% to 66% reported being likely to offer a clinically indicated *APOE* or *PS1* test, depending on whether the patient was symptomatic or not and family history.[34] A survey of 882 physicians similarly found mixed views of predictive genetic testing to identify increased risk for breast or colorectal cancer in the absence of proven preventive or curative interventions, with only 39% agreeing that such tests should be offered.[21] This finding is understandable, given what physicians perceive to be the risks of anxiety and insurance or employment discrimination that such information may cause.[33,35–37]

Provider Information Avoidance and Interest in Receiving Their Own Clinical Whole Exome Sequencing Results

With the expectation that clinicians' experiences with genetic testing and personal preferences in the WES context may color their professional attitudes and opinions, we measured PCPs' preferences for receiving their own genetic results in 2 ways. First, we administered a 2-item scale designed to measure information avoidance (IA).[38] These items, tailored to a genetic health context, asked clinicians to report on a 7-point scale the extent to which they agree that "I would avoid learning about genetic information that could be important to my health (and the health of my family members)" and "Even if it will upset me, I want to know about genetic information that could be important to my health (and the health of my family members)." Geisinger clinicians' reported IA levels were unequivocally low (after reverse scoring the second item) (mean = 2.20 out of 7 possible points; SD = 1.23), with only 5% of all participants scoring above the neutral scale midpoint ("neither agree nor disagree"). The providers also scored substantially lower on IA than a previous sample we collected of 1605 laypeople (paid online workers recruited via Amazon Mechanical Turk) who completed the same 2-item scale (mean = 3.22; SD = 0.92), $t(1,814) = 15.30$, $P<.001$, with a large effect in standard deviation units ($d = 0.83$). A substantial majority of Geisinger providers therefore reported at least some level of agreement that they would choose to learn genetic health information about themselves. As some evidence of behavioral validation for this measure, we did observe a reliable positive correlation over all participants between information seeking (disagreement with the IA scale items) and participants' previous personal participation in any kind of genetic test ($r = 0.21$; $P<.001$). There was no such correlation between participants' self-reported IA scale score and whether they had referred a patient for, ordered, or returned a genetic test result ($r = 0.07$; $P = .135$). We note that any correlations between this measure and others should be treated with caution, given the restricted range on the scale.

As a second measure of preferences regarding WES screening, we asked, "If you were a Geisinger patient, would you choose to learn this information about yourself?" (response options included definitely yes, probably yes, probably not, and definitely not). Whereas the IA scale items were designed to measure preferences for any genetic health information, this item was specifically tailored to Geisinger's recently launched WES screening program. Clinicians expressed a high degree of willingness to learn actionable genetic health information in a WES context (mean = 3.00 out of 4.00; SD = 0.88), regardless of their professional position as an MD, PA, or NP (mean = 3.02; SD = 0.86) or nurse (mean = 2.98; SD = 0.90).

Primary Care Provider Perceptions of Population Genomic Screening

Outside of the carrier screening context, little is known about providers' attitudes toward population genetic/omic screening for actionable variants. A small survey of health care providers found that 48% of all respondents said that they would be willing to offer genetic testing for ovarian cancer risk to all their adult female patients. Broken down by specialty, clinical geneticists were the least likely to be willing to offer such population genetic screening (18%), oncologists were the most likely to be willing (69%), and general practitioners fell somewhere in between (50%).[39] Our providers' indications that they would choose to learn their own clinical WES results (86% choosing probably yes or definitely yes) and, especially, their perception that a hypothetical Geisinger patient who chooses to undergo clinical WES made the right choice (92% stating that the information seeking patient made the right choice; 59% stating that the information avoidant patient made the wrong choice) could be interpreted as proxy measures of providers' support for the clinical WES program.

Our survey measured support more directly, but qualitatively, by inviting respondents to answer an optional open-ended question soliciting their views of the clinical WES program. Fifty-three respondents (12.4% of our sample) provided responses. Consistent with a quantitative study conducted by Hann and colleagues,[39] comments among Geisinger PCPs were about evenly split between enthusiastic and cautious. Enthusiastic respondents:

- Emphasized the benefits of being proactive instead of reactive in health care
- Relayed that patients had expressed interest
- Indicated their own intention to undergo clinical WES testing
- Expressed the view that population genomic screening is part of medicine's inevitable future
- Urged that clinical WES be offered routinely at all Geisinger clinics
- Suggested that patients be incentivized to have the test done as part of preventive medicine

Cautious respondents noted:

- The risk of insurance discrimination
- The need for provider education (about the implications of WES results, how to counsel patients, and how to consent patients for WES testing)
- Their perception that patients are insufficiently educated (to make sound decisions about clinical WES testing, appreciate the limitations and the probabilistic nature of the test, and appreciate the life-altering nature of some preventive measures, eg, prophylactic mastectomies) and that strong educational materials or counseling are needed
- The difficulties of discussing genetic testing during a short primary care visit
- Their uncertainty about data privacy and ownership and a lack of trust in medical and insurance institutions
- That acting on a genotype without a phenotypic presentation may lead to overtreating patients and should be pursued only as part of a clinical trial
- Their belief that population genomic screening is less important than other Geisinger priorities

Finally, our survey explored the possibility that participants' physical work location might be associated with any of the measures we have discussed, hypothesizing that proximity to Geisinger's headquarters and the epicenter of its genomics programs—Geisinger Medical Center in Danville, Pennsylvania—might influence attitudes. Participants reported the region of their primary work location—Geisinger Medical Center, somewhere else in Danville, Pennsylvania, or somewhere in Pennsylvania other than Danville (we excluded 33 participants who reported their location as other). One relationship did emerge: PCPs closer to the epicenter of genomics were more likely to have ordered a test, referred a patient, or returned a result ($r = 0.21$; $P<.001$). We observed no reliable correlation between physical proximity to genomics operations at Geisinger and any other variables collected in this survey (all Pearson r values < 0.07), including the above proxy measures of support for clinical WES, genetics training, personal or professional experience with genetics, ordering and referral behavior, and comfort discussing genetics with patients.

PROVIDER AND LAY PERCEPTIONS OF NUDGING CASCADE TESTING

The population health impact of ascertaining at-risk individuals for medically actionable genetic variants is greatest—and cost-effective—when multiple family members are found to carry the same variant.[40] At Geisinger, as in many other health systems, variant-positive patients are provided with family letters to distribute to at-risk relatives. These letters explain relatives' risk and invite them to contact the GSC Program to discuss testing. Unfortunately, the uptake of so-called cascade testing remains low. In the cancer context, studies have found that only about one-half of at-risk first-degree relatives are tested.[41,42] At Geisinger, across all relevant conditions, we estimate uptake to be even lower: around 10%. Lightweight behavioral interventions (nudges) designed to ease decision-making paths without restricting choice or significantly altering financial costs or incentives have the potential to increase uptake, but may be objectionable to patients and/or providers.[43]

A variety of stakeholders were engaged using quantitative and qualitative methods to elicit attitudes toward 2 ways of nudging cascade counseling and possible testing through family letters. The first nudge adds to the family letter social information about what others have chosen to do in similar situations combined with a photo and a brief story about a Geisinger patient who was happy with her decision to get tested.[44] The second nudge involves changing the default option for making a follow-up appointment by notifying the decision maker that an automatic appointment has already been scheduled for them with the GSC Program (and that they can cancel, miss, or reschedule this appointment at no cost to themselves or others).[45] After reading a brief description of this cascade testing framework, an explanation of the nature and purpose of the nudges, and (in most cases) a version of the family letter, we asked participants to answer the question, "How ethically appropriate is it to use [social information]/[an automatic appointment] to increase genetic health screening for medically actionable results in at-risk family members?" (5 options, ranging from 1 [very ethically inappropriate] to 5 [very ethically appropriate] with a neutral midpoint).

Support was mixed for these 2 approaches to nudging testing uptake (**Fig. 2**). The social information nudge was perceived as just above the scale midpoint in ethical appropriateness and perceived ethical appropriateness did not differ

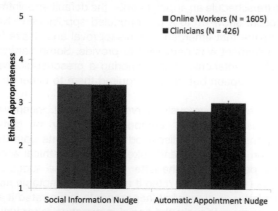

Fig. 2. Perceived ethical appropriateness of 2 nudges designed to increase testing uptake in at-risk populations. Larger values indicate greater rated ethical appropriateness. Error bars show ± 1 standard error of the mean.

between laypeople (mean, 3.43; SD, 1.19) and clinicians (mean = 3.42; SD = 1.16), $t(2,029) = 0.12$, $P = .91$, with a near-zero effect size ($d = 0.01$). The automatic appointment nudge was rated just below the scale midpoint. Here, however, clinicians perceived the nudge to be more ethically appropriate (mean = 3.00; SD = 1.24) than did laypeople (mean = 2.80; SD = 1.24), $t(2,029) = 6.32$, $P<.001$, with a small effect size ($d = 0.34$).

After exploring relationships among measures, we noted one tentative yet interesting potential result. In the full provider sample, the more information-seeking a participant was (as measured by the IA scale), the more ethically appropriate they viewed the social information ($r = 0.239$; $P<.001$) and automatic appointment ($r = 0.237$; $P<.001$) nudges to be. This result was corroborated when considering participants' answer to the question about the clinical WES program for actionable results, "If you were a Geisinger patient, would you choose to learn this information about yourself?" (social information nudge, $r = 0.23$; $P<.001$; automatic appointment nudge, $r = 0.20$; $P = .005$). This relationship replicated for the social information nudge in 1605 online workers ($r = -0.11$; $P<.001$), but did not replicate for the automatic appointment nudge ($r = 0.02$; $P = .42$). This exploratory and preliminary result suggested that the sample of Geisinger clinicians (and to some extent, a large sample of laypeople) may base their ethical judgments of nudges in precision medicine on their own preferences to seek or receive information about themselves (or vice versa; this relationship is merely correlational).

Two small studies were conducted to better understand perceived appropriateness of cascade testing nudges. First, we conducted a focus group (N = 17) of Geisinger patients diverse in sex, educational attainment, age, self-reported health literacy, first- or second-hand experience with cancer, and biobank enrollment and variant-positive status. Participants were compensated with a $15 gift card. After reading the standard family letter and a letter containing a social information nudge, participants found the letter containing a social information nudge to be more engaging and effective in capturing the reader's attention.

To ensure that participants would be willing to tell us that a letter was not ethically appropriate, we asked them to read and consider the default appointment letter. Although recipients would retain the same 2 options they have with either the standard or the social information nudge letter—ignore the letter without penalty or contact the genomics team to (re)schedule an appointment—the default appointment letter would provide a third option: show up to a prescheduled appointment. Nevertheless, the strong dominant theme that emerged was disapproval and desire for more control than a default appointment was perceived to provide. Some participants explained that, given cultural expectations, simply ignoring a prescheduled appointment did not feel like a genuine option but, rather, required them to either show up or call to reschedule or cancel.

Second, our survey anonymously surveyed (without incentive) members of Geisinger's genomics community, composed primarily of genetic counselors (N = 24; 43% response rate). We displayed to respondents both the standard and the social information nudge letter and asked about the ethical acceptability of the latter. Seventy-nine percent rated the letter containing the nudge as somewhat or very acceptable, 4% (1 respondent) rated it as neither acceptable nor unacceptable, and 17% rated the letter as somewhat inappropriate (none rated it as very inappropriate). Ninety-two percent thought the social information letter would be effective. Finally, when asked which of the 2 letters they overall preferred, only 30% chose the standard letter.

SUMMARY AND LIMITATIONS

Geisinger PCPs seem to have modestly more genetics training and ordering and referral experience than other surveyed clinicians. However, like other surveyed providers, Geisinger PCPs reported generally low levels of comfort with answering patients' questions about their risk for inherited. Clinicians stated high levels of willingness to undergo population genomic screening themselves, characterized hypothetical patients who chose to do so as having made the right choice, and, when asked to comment on Geisinger's new clinical WES program, were frequently positive, although several respondents raised concerns about insurance discrimination, false positives, privacy, and other risks. Finally, attitudes were mixed toward the ethical appropriateness of nudges designed to increase testing uptake for actionable results in an at-risk population, though a passive social information nudge was generally preferred to a more direct automatic appointment nudge, which may be viewed as restricting autonomy.

These results are subject to several limitations. We collected data anonymously and were thus unable to test for potential relationships between our primary measures and participants' specialties or demographic characteristics. Owing to our relatively low response rate and our method of recruiting respondents by mass email, our results may not be representative of the Geisinger PCP population as a whole. Finally, the analyses we conducted were run in an exploratory fashion after all data were collected and our results should therefore be treated as exploratory and not necessarily as confirmatory.

The Geisinger survey's results are consistent with those of prior surveys that find that primary care clinicians lack confidence in their knowledge of genetics and in their ability to discuss genetic testing options and results with patients. Some previous work has measured providers' comprehension of genetics and found that their lack of confidence is often warranted. Given patients' increasing access to genetic information in clinical, research, and direct-to-consumer settings, and the willingness of many primary care patients to participate in screening programs,[46] we encourage health systems to provide more opportunities for CME about the broad importance of genetics/omics to common, complex diseases and for primary care clinicians to take advantage of those opportunities. At the same time, we note that at Geisinger, integrating genomics into health care has been successful despite its primary care clinicians' moderately low levels of confidence and only slightly above average ordering and referral experience. Rather than attempting to convert primary care clinicians into medical geneticists, Geisinger's gene-specific, just-in-time clinician educational modules and its small core of 2 or 3 genetic counselors devoted full time to counseling variant-positive patients and their at-risk relatives—and not any unusual experience, confidence, or expertise among its providers—has likely enabled Geisinger to successfully integrate population genomic screening into primary care. Indeed, a more significant obstacle to this integration may be one that is not at all unique to genomics. PCPs will play a pivotal role in offering population genomic screening to patients—and, for variant-positive patients, in encouraging adherence to recommended risk management and cascade testing of at-risk relatives. But there is a dizzying array of other clinical priorities competing for PCPs' already limited time and attention. It is here that clinicians' limited knowledge, experience, and confidence with respect to genetics might pose a threat to integration by biasing them to inappropriately prioritize care gaps they feel most comfortable with. Broad education, confidence-building exposure to primary care settings that have successfully integrated genomics, and nudging both PCPs and patients to begin conversations about genetic risk may all help clinicians to appropriately triage population genomic screening, cascade testing, and adherence to recommended risk management measures.

ACKNOWLEDGMENTS

The authors would like to thank Anh Huynh for research assistance and Dr David Rolston for administering the PCP survey. Survey items and dataset are available at https://osf.io/94esz/. Survey preregistration and detailed reporting of the experimental manipulation are available at https://osf.io/nz6ud/.

REFERENCES

1. Carey DJ, Fetterolf SN, Davis FD, et al. The Geisinger MyCode community health initiative: an electronic health record–linked biobank for precision medicine research. Genet Med 2016;18:906–13.

2. Dewey FE, Murray MF, Overton JD, et al. Distribution and clinical impact of functional variants in 50,726 whole-exome sequences from the DiscoverEHR study. Science 2016;354:1534–6.

3. Faucett WA, Davis FD. How Geisinger made the case for an institutional duty to return genomic results to biobank participants. Appl Transl Genom 2016;8:33–5.

4. Schwartz MLB, McCormick CZ, Lazzeri AL, et al. A model for genome-first care: returning secondary genomics findings to participants and their healthcare providers in a large research cohort. Am J Hum Genet 2018;103:328–37.

5. Geisinger. MyCode scorecard. 2019. Available at: https://www.geisinger.org/-/media/OneGeisinger/pdfs/ghs/research/mycode/mycode-scorecard-feb-2019.pdf?la=en. Accessed March 1, 2019.

6. CDC. Office of Public Health Genomics—Genomic Tests and Family History by Levels of Evidence. 2014. Available at: https://phgkb.cdc.gov/PHGKB/topicStartPage.action. Accessed September 16, 2018.

7. Geisinger. MyCode results reported. 2019. Available at: https://www.geisinger.org/-/media/OneGeisinger/pdfs/ghs/research/mycode/mycode-results-feb-2019.pdf?la=en. Accessed March 1, 2019.

8. Manickam K, Buchanan AH, Schwartz MLB, et al. Exome sequencing-based screening for BRCA1/2 expected pathogenic variants among adult biobank participants. JAMA Netw Open 2018;1:e182140.

9. Buchanan AH, Manickam K, Meyer MN, et al. Early cancer diagnoses through BRCA1/2 screening of unselected adult biobank participants. Genet Med 2018; 20:554–8.

10. Andrews M. What if your doctor offered genetic testing as a way to keep you healthy? Washington Post. 2018. Available at: https://www.washingtonpost.com/national/health-science/what-if-your-doctor-offered-genetic-testing-as-a-way-to-keep-you-healthy/2018/05/25/84b69238-5dd5-11e8-a4a4-c070ef53f315_story.html?noredirect=on&utm_term=.688d14a48f84. Accessed February 15, 2019.

11. Willard HF, Feinberg DT, Ledbetter DH. How Geisinger is using gene screening to prevent disease. Harv Bus Rev 2018. Available at: https://hbr.org/2018/03/how-geisinger-is-using-gene-screening-to-prevent-disease. Accessed May 1, 2019.

12. Stark Z, Dolman L, Manolio TA, et al. Integrating genomics into healthcare: a global responsibility. Am J Hum Genet 2019;104:13–20.

13. National Academies of Sciences, Engineering, and Medicine (NASEM). Implementing and evaluating genomic screening programs in health care systems: proceedings of a workshop. Washington, DC: The National Academies Press; 2018.

14. Emery J, Watson E, Rose P, et al. A systematic review of the literature exploring the role of primary care in genetic services. Fam Pract 1999;16:426–45.
15. Meyer MN, Heck PR, Holtzman GS, et al. Objecting to experiments that compare two unobjectionable policies or treatments. Proc Natl Acad Sci U S A 2019; 116(22):10723–8.
16. Calzone KA, Jenkins J, Yates J, et al. Survey of nursing integration of genomics into nursing practice. J Nurs Scholarsh 2012;44:428–36.
17. Calzone KA, Jenkins J, Culp S, et al. National nursing workforce survey of nursing attitudes, knowledge and practice in genomics. Per Med 2013;10. https://doi.org/10.2217/pme.13.64.
18. Williams JK, Feero WG, Veenstra DL, et al. Considerations in initiating genomic screening programs in health care systems. Nurs Outlook 2018. https://doi.org/10.1016/j.outlook.2018.06.008.
19. Nippert I, Harris HJ, Julian-Reynier C, et al. Confidence of primary care physicians in their ability to carry out basic medical genetic tasks—a European survey in five countries—Part 1. J Community Genet 2010;2:1–11.
20. Cohn J, Blazey W, Tegay D, et al. Physician risk assessment knowledge regarding BRCA genetics testing. J Cancer Educ 2015;30:573–9.
21. Marzuillo C, De Vito C, Boccia S, et al. Knowledge, attitudes and behavior of physicians regarding predictive genetic tests for breast and colorectal cancer. Prev Med 2013;57(5):477–82.
22. Shields AE, Burke W, Levy DE. Differential use of available genetic tests among primary care physicians in the United States: results of a national survey. Genet Med 2008;10:404–14.
23. Coleman B, Calzone KA, Jenkins J, et al. Multi-ethnic minority nurses' knowledge and practice of genetics and genomics. J Nurs Scholarsh 2014;46:235–44.
24. Bellcross CA, Kolor K, Goddard KA, et al. Awareness and utilization of BRCA1/2 testing among U.S. primary care physicians. Am J Prev Med 2011;40(1):61–6.
25. Cox SL, Zlot AI, Silvey K, et al. Patterns of cancer genetic testing: a randomized survey of Oregon clinicians. J Cancer Epidemiol 2012;2012:1–11.
26. Sifri R, Myers R, Hyslop T, et al. Use of cancer susceptibility testing among primary care physicians. Clin Genet 2003;64:355–60.
27. Acton RT, Burst NM, Casebeer L, et al. Knowledge, attitudes and behaviors of Alabama's primary care physicians regarding cancer genetics. Acad Med 2000;75:850–2.
28. Klitzman R, Chung W, Marder K, et al. Attitudes and practices among internists concerning genetic testing. J Genet Couns 2013;22:90–100.
29. Mainous AG III, Johnson SP, Chirina S, et al. Academic family physicians' perception of genetic testing and integration into practice: a CERA study. Fam Med 2013;45(4):257–62.
30. Fry A, Campbell H, Gudmundsdottir H, et al. GPs' views on their role in cancer genetics services and current practice. Fam Pract 1999;16:468–74.
31. Rinke ML, Mikat-Stevens N, Saul R, et al. Genetic services and attitudes in primary care pediatrics. Am J Med Genet 2013;164A:449–55.
32. Heck PR, Meyer MM. Information avoidance in genetic health: perceptions, norms, and preferences. Soc Cognit 2019;37(3):266–93.
33. Watson EK, Shickle D, Qureshi N, et al. The 'new genetics' and primary care: GPs' views on their role and their educational needs. Fam Pract 1999;16(4):420–5.

34. Chase GA, Geller G, Havstad SL, et al. Physicians' propensity to offer genetic testing for Alzheimer's disease: results from a survey. Genet Med 2002;4: 297–303.
35. Falahee M, Simons G, Raza K, et al. Healthcare professionals' perceptions of risk in the context of genetic testing for the prediction of chronic disease: a qualitative metasynthesis. J Risk Res 2016;21(2):1–38.
36. Freedman AN, Wideroff L, Olson L, et al. US physicians' attitudes toward genetic testing for cancer susceptibility. Am J Med Genet 2003;120:63–71.
37. Chowdhury S, Dent T, Pashayan N, et al. Incorporating genomics into breast and prostate cancer screening: assessing the implications. Genet Med 2013;15(6): 423–32.
38. Howell JL, Shepperd JA. Establishing an information avoidance scale. Psychol Assess 2016;28(12):1–14.
39. Hann KE, Fraser L, Side L, et al. Health care professionals' attitudes towards population-based genetic testing and risk stratification for ovarian cancer: a cross-sectional survey. BMC Womens Health 2017;17:132.
40. Ladabaum U, Wang G, Terdiman J, et al. Strategies to identify the Lynch syndrome among patients with colorectal cancer: a cost-effectiveness analysis. Ann Intern Med 2011;155:69–79.
41. Sharaf RN, Myer P, Stave CD, et al. Uptake of genetic testing by relatives of lynch syndrome probands: a systematic review. Clin Gastroenterol Hepatol 2013;11: 1093–100.
42. Caswell-Jin JL, Zimmer AD, Stedden W, et al. Cascade genetic testing of relatives for hereditary cancer risk: results of an online initiative. J Natl Cancer Inst 2019;111:95–8.
43. Thaler RH, Sunstein CR. Nudge: improving decisions about health, wealth, and happiness. New York: Penguin; 2009.
44. Cialdini RB. Harnessing the science of persuasion. Harv Bus Rev 2001;79:72–81.
45. Johnson EJ, Goldstein D. Do defaults save lives? Science 2003;302:1338–9.
46. Hulick P, Dunnenberger H, Neben C, et al. Implementation of hereditary cancer genetic testing in the primary care setting. Poster presented at: ACMG Annual Clinical Genetics Meeting; 2019 Apr 2–6; Seattle, WA. Available at: https://static.getcolor.com/pdfs/research/2019_ACMG_Peter_J_Hulick.pdf. Accessed May 1, 2019.

UNITED STATES POSTAL SERVICE ® Statement of Ownership, Management, and Circulation (All Periodicals Publications Except Requester Publications)

1. Publication Title	2. Publication Number	3. Filing Date
MEDICAL CLINICS IN NORTH AMERICA	337 – 340	9/18/2019

4. Issue Frequency	5. Number of Issues Published Annually	6. Annual Subscription Price
JAN, MAR, MAY, JUL, SEP, NOV	6	$284.00

7. Complete Mailing Address of Known Office of Publication *(Not printer) (Street, city, county, state, and ZIP+4®)*

ELSEVIER INC.
230 Park Avenue, Suite 800
New York, NY 10169

Contact Person
STEPHEN R. BUSHING

Telephone *(Include area code)*
215-239-3688

8. Complete Mailing Address of Headquarters or General Business Office of Publisher *(Not printer)*

ELSEVIER INC.
230 Park Avenue, Suite 800
New York, NY 10169

9. Full Names and Complete Mailing Addresses of Publisher, Editor, and Managing Editor *(Do not leave blank)*

Publisher *(Name and complete mailing address)*

TAYLOR BALL, ELSEVIER INC.
1600 JOHN F KENNEDY BLVD. SUITE 1800
PHILADELPHIA, PA 19103-2899

Editor *(Name and complete mailing address)*

KATERINA HEIDHAUSEN, ELSEVIER INC.
1600 JOHN F KENNEDY BLVD. SUITE 1800
PHILADELPHIA, PA 19103-2899

Managing Editor *(Name and complete mailing address)*

PATRICK MANLEY, ELSEVIER INC.
1600 JOHN F KENNEDY BLVD. SUITE 1800
PHILADELPHIA, PA 19103-2899

10. Owner *(Do not leave blank. If the publication is owned by a corporation, give the name and address of the corporation immediately followed by the names and addresses of all stockholders owning or holding 1 percent or more of the total amount of stock. If not owned by a corporation, give the names and addresses of the individual owners. If owned by a partnership or other unincorporated firm, give its name and address as well as those of each individual owner. If the publication is published by a nonprofit organization, give its name and address.)*

Full Name	Complete Mailing Address
WHOLLY OWNED SUBSIDIARY OF REED/ELSEVIER, US HOLDINGS	1600 JOHN F KENNEDY BLVD. SUITE 1800 PHILADELPHIA, PA 19103-2899

11. Known Bondholders, Mortgagees, and Other Security Holders Owning or Holding 1 Percent or More of Total Amount of Bonds, Mortgages, or Other Securities. If none, check box ► ☐ None

Full Name	Complete Mailing Address
N/A	

12. Tax Status *(For completion by nonprofit organizations authorized to mail at nonprofit rates) (Check one)*
The purpose, function, and nonprofit status of this organization and the exempt status for federal income tax purposes:
☒ Has Not Changed During Preceding 12 Months
☐ Has Changed During Preceding 12 Months *(Publisher must submit explanation of change with this statement)*

PS Form 3526, July 2014 *(Page 1 of 4 (see instructions page 4))* PSN: 7530-01-000-9931 PRIVACY NOTICE: See our privacy policy on www.usps.com.

13. Publication Title		14. Issue Date for Circulation Data Below
MEDICAL CLINICS IN NORTH AMERICA		JULY 2019

15. Extent and Nature of Circulation		Average No. Copies Each Issue During Preceding 12 Months	No. Copies of Single Issue Published Nearest to Filing Date
a. Total Number of Copies *(Net press run)*		437	496
b. Paid Circulation (By Mail and Outside the Mail)	(1) Mailed Outside-County Paid Subscriptions Stated on PS Form 3541 (Include paid distribution above nominal rate, advertiser's proof copies, and exchange copies)	230	277
	(2) Mailed In-County Paid Subscriptions Stated on PS Form 3541 (Include paid distribution above nominal rate, advertiser's proof copies, and exchange copies)	0	0
	(3) Paid Distribution Outside the Mails Including Sales Through Dealers and Carriers, Street Vendors, Counter Sales, and Other Paid Distribution Outside USPS®	119	165
	(4) Paid Distribution by Other Classes of Mail Through the USPS (e.g., First-Class Mail®)	0	0
c. Total Paid Distribution *(Sum of 15b (1), (2), (3), and (4))* ►		349	442
d. Free or Nominal Rate Distribution (By Mail and Outside the Mail)	(1) Free or Nominal Rate Outside-County Copies included on PS Form 3541	73	35
	(2) Free or Nominal Rate In-County Copies Included on PS Form 3541	0	0
	(3) Free or Nominal Rate Copies Mailed at Other Classes Through the USPS (e.g., First-Class Mail)	0	0
	(4) Free or Nominal Rate Distribution Outside the Mail (Carriers or other means)	0	0
e. Total Free or Nominal Rate Distribution *(Sum of 15d (1), (2), (3) and (4))* ►		73	35
f. Total Distribution *(Sum of 15c and 15e)* ►		422	477
g. Copies not Distributed *(See Instructions to Publishers #4 (page #3))* ►		15	19
h. Total *(Sum of 15f and g)* ►		437	496
i. Percent Paid *(15c divided by 15f times 100)* ►		82.7%	92.66%

* If you are claiming electronic copies, go to line 16 on page 3. If you are not claiming electronic copies, skip to line 17 on page 3.

16. Electronic Copy Circulation	Average No. Copies Each Issue During Preceding 12 Months	No. Copies of Single Issue Published Nearest to Filing Date
a. Paid Electronic Copies ►		
b. Total Paid Print Copies (Line 15c) + Paid Electronic Copies (Line 16a) ►		
c. Total Print Distribution (Line 15f) + Paid Electronic Copies (Line 16a) ►		
d. Percent Paid (Both Print & Electronic Copies) (16b divided by 16c × 100) ►		

☒ I certify that 50% of all my distributed copies (electronic and print) are paid above a nominal price.

17. Publication of Statement of Ownership

☒ If the publication is a general publication, publication of this statement is required. Will be printed in the NOVEMBER 2019 issue of this publication.   ☐ Publication not required.

18. Signature and Title of Editor, Publisher, Business Manager, or Owner		Date
STEPHEN R. BUSHING - INVENTORY DISTRIBUTION CONTROL MANAGER	*Stephen R. Bushing*	9/18/2019

I certify that all information furnished on this form is true and complete. I understand that anyone who furnishes false or misleading information on this form or who omits material or information requested on the form may be subject to criminal sanctions (including fines and imprisonment) and/or civil sanctions (including civil penalties).

PS Form 3526, July 2014 *(Page 3 of 4)* PRIVACY NOTICE: See our privacy policy on www.usps.com

Moving?

Make sure your subscription moves with you!

To notify us of your new address, find your **Clinics Account Number** (located on your mailing label above your name), and contact customer service at:

Email: journalscustomerservice-usa@elsevier.com

800-654-2452 (subscribers in the U.S. & Canada)
314-447-8871 (subscribers outside of the U.S. & Canada)

Fax number: 314-447-8029

Elsevier Health Sciences Division
Subscription Customer Service
3251 Riverport Lane
Maryland Heights, MO 63043

*To ensure uninterrupted delivery of your subscription, please notify us at least 4 weeks in advance of move.

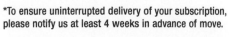

Moving?

Make sure your subscription moves with you!

To notify us of your new address, find your Clinics Account Number (located on your mailing label above your name), and contact customer service at:

Email: journalscustomerservice-usa@elsevier.com

800-654-2452 (subscribers in the U.S. & Canada)
314-447-8871 (subscribers outside of the U.S. & Canada)

Fax number: 314-447-8029

Elsevier Health Sciences Division
Subscription Customer Service
3251 Riverport Lane
Maryland Heights, MO 63043

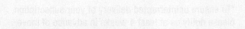

Printed and bound by CPI Group (UK) Ltd, Croydon, CR0 4YY

03/10/2024

01040400-0010